Contents

The World Drug Situation

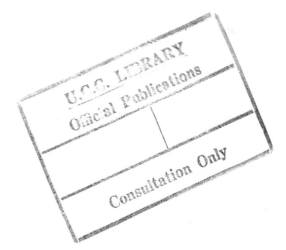
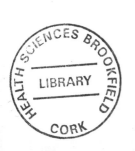

WORLD HEALTH ORGANIZATION
GENEVA
1988

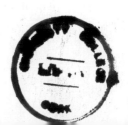

PRINTED IN SWITZERLAND

88/7578 – IAM – 5500

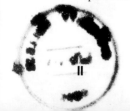

Preface

In 1977 the World Health Organization published the first model list of essential drugs, and in 1981 the WHO Action Programme on Essential Drugs was launched. Since then a large number of countries have adopted an essential drugs policy. The progress achieved in those countries has been described in many WHO reports, but no systematic description of the drug situation at global and national levels in the public and private sectors has been undertaken in recent years. The Conference of Experts on the Rational Use of Drugs held under the auspices of the World Health Organization in Nairobi in 1985[1] acknowledged the need for more information on the drug situation at the global and national levels, and requested WHO to provide this information as part of its revised drug strategy.

The present report responds to that request. It should be regarded as a baseline survey carried out with limited resources, and will be updated at regular intervals.

A set of indicators has been selected to monitor progress by countries towards attaining the objectives of a national drug policy.[2] These objectives can be summarized as follows:

— to make effective, safe, low-cost drugs available to meet the needs of the entire population (essential drugs);

— to ensure that drugs are used rationally;

— to develop, where economically and technically feasible, national pharmaceutical production that supports economic growth and the overall development strategy of the country.

Approaches and strategies differ greatly. No single drug policy is suitable for all countries, given the differences in manpower, research, financial resources, and other characteristics. For this reason the present report attempts mainly to identify outputs; where strategies are described, it is by way of example.

The report has been synthesized from a large number of government and other country reports. National and international publications, including trade publications, have been scrutinized, and data have been collected through discussions with nationals working in the field and with WHO staff members at country and regional level. The synthesis of such a large

---

[1] *The rational use of drugs. Report of the Conference of Experts, Nairobi, 25-29 November 1985.* Geneva, World Health Organization, 1987.

[2] *Guidelines for developing national drug policies.* Geneva, World Health Organization, 1988.

amount of information presents special problems. Careful selection and distillation of material are required and it is possible that important developments taking place at country level have been omitted. At best, such a synthesis can indicate only the most significant trends and areas of progress and analyse the principal issues and obstacles faced by WHO Member States in implementing their national drug policy.

The report is divided into two parts. The first part describes the situation of demand and supply at global level, in other words the production and consumption of drugs in the world and their geographical distribution. The second part describes the situation in individual countries and the steps taken to achieve the objectives listed above. No baseline survey was available and, where feasible, emphasis has been put on trends and progress.

*
* *

Special mention should be made of Ms P. Brudon Jakobowicz, of WHO's Action Programme on Essential Drugs, for her major contribution to the preparation of this report.

PART I

The international scene

Introduction

Even in the remotest areas of the world people consume modern drugs. These drugs are now part of the armamentarium of medical practitioners and healers at every level and are universally perceived to have — and often do have — powerful effects. They form part of a specific rational approach to treatment that has spread throughout the world.

The first part of this report concentrates on the broad aspects — qualitative as well as quantitative — of drug consumption, production, and trade. The intention is to provide an overview of the current drug situation throughout the world which will serve as a background to the more detailed descriptions given in the second part of the report. It is not meant to be an exhaustive analysis of the situation, which would itself require a full report. It will be continuously updated in the data bank of the WHO Action Programme on Essential Drugs.

This first part is divided into three chapters. Chapter 1 briefly discusses traditional medicines, as they are an important form of treatment. Chapter 2 assesses drug consumption in the world, the geographical distribution of consumption in developed and developing countries, consumption patterns, and the use of drugs. Chapter 3 describes trends in world production and trade and includes an overview of drug suppliers — national producers in developing countries, producers of generic drugs, and the research-based pharmaceutical industry.

Chapter 1

Traditional medicine

For thousands of years mankind has employed a variety of ways of dealing with disease. In all societies there have been remedies and people to advise on how to deal with disease and its consequences. For vast numbers of people, traditional medicine is still the only form of treatment available to them. Moreover, even in countries where the governments have succeeded in making modern health care available to the population, people continue to seek traditional treatment. Sometimes this traditional treatment is more expensive than that provided by the government, but the services and advice of indigenous practitioners are valued because they are offered in terms that patients can understand and in the context of cultural values and practices that are shared by patients and healers alike. The traditional healer takes the time to find out about the patient's family history and problems and on that basis suggests rituals, sacrifices, herbal medicines, and other forms of treatment. In contrast to "Western" medicine, the traditional healer involves the family and other people from the patient's circle of friends and relatives in both treatment of the disease and responsibility for it. Traditional healers treat body, mind, and social relations as an indivisible unit. This holistic approach is, most of all, the special characteristic of systems of traditional medicine.

Allopathic medicine spread in the Third World during the colonial period, but it was generally limited to a very small group, usually white people based in the cities; in the rural areas traditional medicine largely remained the only source of treatment. The achievement of independence for many countries meant an extension of allopathic medicine into the rural areas where the majority of people live. In fact, people generally establish some sort of division of work between the two systems. Many studies have shown that people are essentially pragmatic; they make their initial choice of treatment on the basis of their perception of the cause of the illness, whether natural or supernatural. If the treatment does not work they shift easily to a conceptually different treatment. In some cultures patients with acute diseases are brought for allopathic treatment and those with chronic diseases for traditional treatment. Very often both systems are used at the same time.

Traditional healers to an increasing extent incorporate modern drugs in their therapies, so as to attract patients. This may be a cause for concern, as these healers have no training in the use of pharmaceuticals, their information regarding drug indications, contraindications, side-effects, etc., being derived from informal non-medical sources or from drug retailers with extremely limited knowledge.

Some governments are trying to make use of the traditional healer's skill in providing psychological and social support for the ill, and a number of studies have suggested that collaboration between folk medicine and modern medicine could increase the efficacy of certain treatments. However, collaboration is not easy, since the contribution of traditional healers to the health and well-being of patients has for too long been ridiculed or ignored by modern medical practitioners. Governments have also appeared to focus more on the potential of herbal remedies than the skills of traditional healers. Many plans have been launched, with scant success, for the industrialized production of medicines from herbal plants in developing countries. More information is needed on the volume of consumption of herbal and other traditional medicines and their efficacy, in view of the extent to which they are used, but such information is extremely difficult to obtain.

Chapter 2

Drug consumption

Global figures

During the past decade the value of world consumption of drugs at current prices has increased dramatically. Whereas in 1976 it amounted to US$ 43 billion,[1,2] in 1985 it reached US$ 94.1 billion, an average annual increase of 9.1% (1).

A similar increase took place at the level of the individual: during the decade the average yearly per capita drug expenditure in the world nearly doubled, from US$ 10.3 in 1976 to US$ 19.4 in 1985 (2).

These figures, however, do not provide a full picture of the world drug situation. For example, they do not reflect the fact that in Mexico, the average consumer spent less of his real income on drugs in 1985 than in 1976: at 1980 prices he spent, on average, 565 pesos on drugs in 1976 and only 547 pesos in 1985. At least three major factors have to be taken into account in assessing the global situation:

(1) the geographical distribution of drug consumption in the world;

(2) the evolution of per capita drug consumption;

(3) monetary factors.

The geographical distribution of drug consumption

One element that global figures do not reflect is the uneven distribution of consumption in the world. In 1976 more than three-quarters of the drugs produced were consumed by the 27% of the world's population living in developed countries.[2]

In 1985, this gap had increased further — the 75% of the world population living in developing countries consumed only 21% of the world's drugs

---

[1] All figures are expressed at the ex-manufacturer price and at the current exchange rate if not otherwise specified. Billion in this report means a thousand million (10⁹).

[2] *Global study of the pharmaceutical industry.* Unpublished UNIDO document, ID/WG.331/6, 1980.

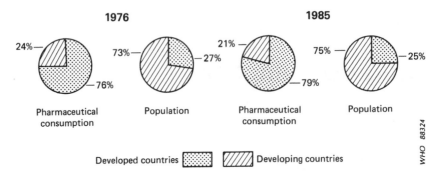

Fig. 1
Geographical distribution of world drug consumption and population, 1976 and 1985.

(Fig. 1).[1] This increasing imbalance is due to the fact that drug consumption grew at an average of 9.6% per year in developed countries, and at only 7.2% in developing countries. In other words, in 1985, 1.2 billion people living in developed countries consumed nearly US$ 75 billion worth of drugs while the remaining 4 billion living in developing countries consumed only US$ 20 billion worth (Table 1).

Table 1.   World consumption of pharmaceuticals by region (US$ billion, ex-manufacturer price)[a]

	1976	1985
North America	8.761	28.141
Western Europe	13.111	22.000
Eastern Europe	6.197	9.600
Japan	4.020	14.038
Oceania	0.480	0.700
Latin America	3.689	5.600
Africa	1.268	2.700
Asia[b]	2.920	6.600
China	2.600	4.700
Total	43.046	94.079

[a] Sources: *Global study of the pharmaceutical industry,* unpublished UNIDO document ID/WG.331/6, 1980; *IMS Marketletter,* 11 August 1986; *Pharmaceutical business opportunities with China,* SCRIP, 1987.

[b] Excluding China and Japan.

_____

[1] *IMS Marketletter,* 11 August 1986, p. 15, UNIDO data bank, and estimates of the WHO secretariat.

Even these figures overstate the availability of pharmaceuticals in certain countries. The twenty largest markets accounted for 73% of world consumption in 1976, and for 80% in 1985. If Eastern Europe is excluded (US$ 6.2 billion in 1976, US$ 9.6 billion in 1985), the twenty largest markets accounted for 87.5% of consumption in 1976, and for 88.5% in 1985. The eight developing countries included in the top twenty together consumed 64% of the drugs available in the developing world in 1985 (Table 2).

Table 2. **The twenty largest drug markets, 1976 and 1985** (excluding Eastern Europe)[a]

1976			1985		
Country	Sales (US$ billion)	% of world market	Country	Sales (US$ billion)	% of world market
USA	7.900	18.3	USA	26.451	28.1
Japan	4.020	9.3	Japan	14.038	14.9
Federal Republic of Germany	3.410	7.9	Federal Republic of Germany	5.995	6.4
France	2.700	6.3	China	4.700	5.0[b]
China	2.600	6.0	France	4.465	4.7
Italy	1.900	4.4	Italy	3.671	3.9
Spain	1.320	3.0	United Kingdom	2.348	2.5
Brazil	1.210	2.8	India	1.775	1.9
United Kingdom	1.030	2.4	Canada	1.690	1.8
Mexico	0.774	1.8	Brazil	1.408	1.5
Canada	0.672	1.6	Spain	1.397	1.5
Argentina	0.654	1.5	Mexico	1.248	1.3
Belgium	0.536	1.2	Argentina	1.211	1.3
India	0.508	1.1	Republic of Korea	1.013	1.1
Australia	0.411	1.0	Egypt	0.707	0.75
Republic of Korea	0.400	0.9	Belgium	0.694	0.70
Sweden	0.400	0.9	Switzerland	0.605	0.65
Netherlands	0.364	0.85	Australia	0.580	0.60
Switzerland	0.330	0.75	Islamic Republic of Iran	0.513	0.55
Venezuela	0.282	0.65	Netherlands	0.506	0.50
Total for top 20 drug markets	31.421	73	Total for top 20 drug markets	75.015	80
Global total	43.046	100	Global total	94.100	100

[a] Sources: *Global study of the pharmaceutical industry.* Unpublished UNIDO document, ID/WG.331/6, 1980; *IMS Marketletter*, 11 August 1986, p. 15.

[b] *Pharmaceutical business opportunities with China*, SCRIP, 1987.

Developed world

In the developed world in 1985 (Fig. 2) the overall picture was different from that of the mid-1970s. Whereas in 1976 Western Europe as a whole was the most important drug market among developed countries, with 41% of the total, in 1985 it accounted for less than one-third of the total for developed countries, expressed in US$. A decrease also took place in Eastern Europe, while Japan and North America increased their share; North America now consumes more than one-third of the total for the developed world.

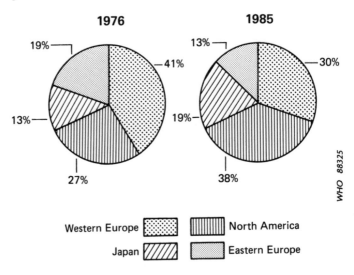

Fig. 2
Drug consumption in developed countries, 1976 and 1985.

These changes in the distribution of consumption cannot be ascribed entirely to changes in consumption patterns, which are relatively stable in the developed countries. A major reason is fluctuation in the currency exchange rate, especially the considerable increase in the value of the US dollar during this period relative to other currencies. In national currency the growth in consumption has in fact been very similar in the United States of America and in the other major developed countries, with the exception of the Federal Republic of Germany and Japan (Table 3). The lower growth rate in those countries is due to a lower rate of inflation during the period 1976–85 and to the strength of their currencies. In other words, except for those two countries, the increase in the amount of national currencies spent on drugs was very similar in most developed countries between 1978 and 1985. In most developed countries people spent a greater percentage of their resources on drugs in 1985 than in 1976. It should be stressed, however, that this percentage remained below 2% of their final consumption (Table 4). It would be useful to determine the kinds of drugs that contributed most to this increase in spending, and what has been their impact on other forms of care, such as hospitalization.

Table 3. Value of drug consumption in 1985 relative to that in 1976 (1976 = 100)[a]

	Value in US$	Value in national currency
France	165	311
Federal Republic of Germany	176	205
Italy	193	346
United Kingdom	228	316
USA	335	335
Japan	349	236

[a] Source: *IMS Marketletter*, 11 August 1986.

Table 4. Share of drug consumption in final consumption[a]

	1976	1985
North America	0.71	1.01
Europe	1.18	1.27
Japan	1.24	1.81
Total	0.96	1.20

[a] Source: *IMS Marketletter*, 11 August 1986; OECD National Accounts 1960–1985, Paris 1987.

The smaller increase in the figures for Europe is a result of the price control policies of some governments. The prices of drugs rose more slowly than those of other consumer goods, whereas in the USA after 1980 price rises by the main companies were well above the rate of inflation.

Developing countries

In developing countries the major change in the geographical distribution of drug consumption in the last ten years has been the large decrease in the Latin American share of total drug consumption (Fig. 3).

11

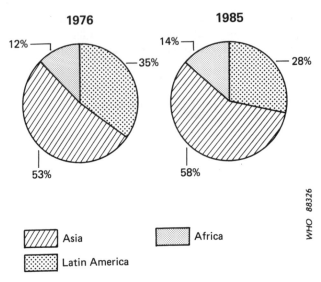

Fig. 3
Drug consumption in developing countries, 1976 and 1985.

There are several reasons for the slower growth in Latin America. The first is price erosion. In terms of the US dollar, over the period 1981–85 the prices of drugs fell in Argentina by 37.6%, in Brazil by 13%, in Chile by 51.7%, in Mexico by 21.5%, and in Venezuela by 52.7% (3). This erosion is due both to the high inflation rate in Latin American countries during this period and to the exchange rate fluctuations and drastic anti-inflationary and other fiscal measures taken by certain Latin American governments. The economic crisis and the related measures taken by governments have also impaired purchasing power in most countries.

Another factor for countries that import the major part of their pharmaceutical consumption is the debt crisis and the lack of hard currency, which have slowed down the overall imports of Latin American countries from an average annual growth rate of 28.5% during 1970–75 to 4.8% during 1975–85 (4).

The evolution of per capita drug consumption

The second element to be taken into account when assessing world drug consumption is per capita drug consumption. As a whole this indicator does not, at least in developing countries and in countries without social security, reflect the consumption of drugs throughout the community; as an average value, it is likely to be far from the extremes. However, it does help to give an idea of the discrepancies that exist between countries, which will be further described in Part II.

Table 5. Value of drug consumption per capita in 1976 and 1985 in developing and developed countries (US$)[a]

	1976	1985	Annual growth rate (%)
Developed countries	29.0	62.1	8.8
Western Europe	34.0	54.5	5.4
North America	36.3	106.3	12.7
Eastern Europe	17.0	24.5	4.1
Japan	35.6	116.3	14.0
Developing countries	3.4	5.4	5.0
Asia	2.4	4.2	6.3
Africa	3.0	4.9	5.7
Latin America	11.2	13.8	2.3
World	10.3	19.4	7.2

[a] Source: *Global study of the pharmaceutical industry*, unpublished UNIDO document, ID/WG.331/6, 1980; *IMS Marketletter*, 11 August 1986; estimates of the WHO secretariat.

The gap in per capita drug consumption between the developed and the developing countries, which was already very considerable in 1976, continued to grow in the subsequent ten years (Table 5). While in terms of value each inhabitant of a developed country consumed on average in 1976 8.5 times as many drugs as an inhabitant of a developing country, in 1985 he consumed drugs costing 11.5 times as much. This worsening of the situation is due to both the slower growth of drug consumption in developing countries and the faster growth of population. Whereas the growth rate of the population in developing countries reached 2.1% per year in the period 1976–85, in developed countries it was less than 0.8%.

The average regional figures do not reflect the differences between countries in the same region. In 1985, for example, as shown in Table 6, Argentina spent US$ 39.6 per capita on drugs, while Brazil spent only US$ 10.3, the United States spent US$ 110.5, and Sweden spent US$ 54.1.

Aggregate expenditure figures also mask the relatively small public sector share of expenditure on pharmaceuticals in most developing countries, in contrast to the large public sector share in many developed countries. Although pharmaceuticals account for 10–35% of ministry of health budgets in developing countries (5), the low allocation to these budgets makes the figure low in absolute terms.

Furthermore, the slow-down in economic growth in the 1980s has led to substantial cutbacks in the health budgets of a number of countries. The

Table 6. Value of drug consumption per capita in individual countries (US$)[a]

	1976		1985
Federal Republic of Germany	55.4	Japan	116.2
Belgium	54.6	USA	110.5
Switzerland	52.1	Federal Republic of Germany	98.2
France	51.0	Switzerland	92.6
Sweden	48.6	France	80.9
USA	36.2	Belgium	70.4
Japan	35.6	Canada	66.5
Italy	34.1	Italy	64.2
Canada	29.1	Sweden	54.1
Netherlands	26.4	United Kingdom	41.4
Argentina	24.7	Argentina	39.6
United Kingdom	18.3	Spain	36.1
Mexico	12.5	Netherlands	34.9
Brazil	10.9	Mexico	15.7
Spain	10.1	Egypt	15.0
Egypt	3.7	Brazil	10.3
China	2.7	China	4.4
India	0.8	India	2.3

[a] Sources: *Global study of the pharmaceutical industry*, Unpublished UNIDO document, ID/WG.331/6, 1980; *IMS Marketletter*, 11 August 1986, p. 15; *Pharmaceutical business opportunities with China*, SCRIP, 1987; and *World population prospects*, New York, UNDIESA, 1986 (Population Studies No. 98).

main source of growth in pharmaceutical consumption has been the private sector (6), where drugs have mostly to be bought by individuals out of their own pocket. Data on this private expenditure are scarce, but it is known that the urban and rural poor consume a disproportionately small share of total national pharmaceutical supplies. This pattern of consumption is reflected in the concentration of pharmaceutical outlets in urban areas, where the purchasing power is higher. More information is required on household expenditure patterns by socioeconomic level in the developing countries. WHO is at present assisting a number of countries in investigating this question.

Some redistribution of public spending on pharmaceuticals in favour of primary health care and underserved groups has been achieved recently by the increasing number of countries that are implementing essential drugs programmes, as described in Part II of this report. In those countries, although consumption in terms of value is still low, resources are being used more efficiently. It has been estimated that coverage with essential drugs in primary health care can be achieved for less than US$ 1 per person per year (7, 8).

Monetary factors

As noted previously, monetary factors — exchange rates and inflation — obscure the picture of the evolution of drug consumption in countries.

In many developing countries people spent more on drugs in 1985 than in 1976. However, this does not necessarily mean that they consumed more. One way to assess whether the volume of drugs consumed per capita has increased is to attempt to correct figures for inflation, by dividing the per capita drug consumption in a national currency by the index of drug prices.[1]

The per capita consumption thus obtained shows that, in terms of volume, the evolution has been very different in different countries. Whereas among European countries the increase was almost the same, it was much greater in North America and Japan. In developing countries, and specifically in Latin America, the per capita consumption remained almost constant during the decade (Table 7).

Table 7.   1985 index of per capita drug consumption (1976 = 100)[a]

Country	Index[b]	Country	Index[b]
Japan	185	Belgium	115
Pakistan	180	Netherlands	110
USA	174	Thailand	105
Canada	161	Brazil	103
Indonesia	152	Algeria	97
Federal Republic of Germany	147	Mexico	96
United Kingdom	136	Philippines	95
France	129	Sweden	92
Switzerland	127	Colombia	82
Italy	119	Nigeria	35

[a] Source: See Table 6.

[b] In national currency and at constant price.

Drug consumption patterns

Consumption patterns can reveal more about the pharmaceutical situation than global figures. A number of publications have discussed at length the inappropriateness of the expensive and often ineffective products consumed in developing countries, and there is a broad consensus that current drug consumption in developing countries is far from being

---

[1] Consumer price indices have been used here as a substitute for drug prices. They suffer from the obvious bias that drug prices in certain countries have not evolved in parallel with prices of other consumer goods.

rational (9). This means that resources are being used for products that are not essential, at a time when a large proportion of the population is without access to even the most basic drugs. In developed countries too, concern has been expressed recently about the rationality of consumption patterns (10-12).

Major therapeutic classes and leading products

Consideration of the world drug consumption by major therapeutic classes shows clearly that the market responds primarily to the needs of the developed countries (Table 8). Between 1975 and 1985, cardiovascular drugs increased their share of the world market from 14% to 18%; a quarter of the new chemical entities introduced between 1982 and 1986 were cardiovascular products; they were followed by psychotropic drugs and anti-inflammatory products (13, 14). In 1975 antimicrobials accounted for 9–15% of consumption in developed countries, and 20–24% in developing countries.[1] Today they still have the largest share of the market in developing countries: 19.2% of total drug sales in 1985 (Table 9). In the United States and Europe they have been overtaken by cardiovascular drugs: roughly 20% of pharmaceutical sales for 1985 in the former and 24% in the latter. Japan is an exception among industrialized countries with anti-infective drugs accounting for nearly 22% of the market, mainly because of the high consumption of expensive antibiotics, mostly cephalosporins.[2]

Table 8. **Percentage of world drug sales for each major therapeutic class**[a]

Therapeutic class	1975	1980	1983	1984	1985
Cardiovascular	14.0	16.1	16.8	17.3	18.1
Anti-infective	17.6	18.0	17.6	17.6	17.1
Internal medicine	15.9	14.6	14.5	14.5	14.6
Analgesics	15.0	13.6	13.5	13.2	12.9
Respiratory	8.5	7.8	7.1	6.9	7.1
Mental health	8.3	7.7	7.1	7.1	6.9
Nutritional	6.7	7.3	7.7	7.6	7.6
Other	14.0	14.9	15.7	15.8	15.7

[a] Source: CAPLIN, D. & GAMBA, J. *Pharmaceuticals strategy paper*, Washington, DC, World Bank, 1985; *SCRIP Yearbook*, 1987.

---

[1] *Global study of the pharmaceutical industry*. Unpublished UNIDO document, ID/WG.331/6, 1980.

[2] This last example shows the limitations of the evaluation of drug consumption in terms of market value. It would be more accurate to evaluate by volume, but no data are available. However, although differences in pricing policy for various therapeutic groups may affect the ranking of therapeutic groups according to market sales, sales can still provide useful pointers to trends.

Table 9. Percentage of drug sales for each major therapeutic class by region (1983 and 1985)[a]

Therapeutic class	USA		Europe		Japan		Rest of the world	
	1983	1985	1983	1985	1983	1985	1983	1985
Cardiovascular	19.1	20.8	22.9	24.3	12.2	13.6	12.9	13.5
Anti-infective	15.1	15.0	16.1	13.8	23.8	21.2	17.8	19.2
Internal medicine	17.4	17.0	11.6	11.9	13.1	13.1	15.7	15.8
Analgesics	11.9	11.5	13.0	13.5	9.5	8.6	16.1	14.6
Respiratory	4.3	4.0	7.6	7.9	3.2	4.6	9.4	9.1
Mental health	9.9	10.4	9.0	8.4	10.3	10.3	3.2	2.7
Nutritional	7.6	6.8	9.1	8.9	12.4	13.5	5.0	5.0
Other	14.7	14.5	10.7	11.3	15.5	15.1	19.9	20.1

[a] Source: *SCRIP Yearbook*, 1987, p. 21.

Analysis of the leading individual products also shows that they cater primarily to the needs of developed countries. In the last ten years the leading products have been mainly for the treatment of ulcers, anxiety, and hypertension (Table 10).

The pattern shows the low effective demand in developing countries for drugs of the highest health priority for the majority of the population, namely, those for tropical infections and parasitic diseases, and the relatively high demand for drugs that do not meet the main needs and are chiefly consumed by a small segment of the population. This situation is exemplified by the fact that H_2 antagonists (anti-ulcer drugs) were among the five leading products in all the regions of the world in 1985.

Drug use

Country-specific data on prescribing patterns and drug use, though extremely scarce, suggest that in developed and developing countries alike, medical personnel, other prescribers, and the public are not rational in their use of drugs. Much has been written on prescribing practices. A study carried out in seven European countries showed marked differences in the utilization of antidiabetic drugs, especially oral preparations. The data available suggest that the incidence of diabetes does not differ as markedly as does drug utilization between countries (*15*). Another comparative study has shown that hospitalized patients in the USA receive twice as many drugs as hospitalized patients in Scotland (*16*). There is also a great variation in Nordic countries in the number of antihypertensives prescribed, a variation that cannot be explained either by differences in morbidity or in the training of or information received by those prescribing (*17*). Comparison of the prescriptions issued in 1985 for the top twenty drugs in five European

Table 10.   Leading products in the world drugs market[a]

		1977		
Brand name	Generic name	Company	Category	Indication
Valium	diazepam	Roche	anxiolytic	anxiety
Aldomet	methyldopa	Merck	hypotensive	hypertension
Keflex	cefalexin	Eli Lilly	antibiotic	infection
Keflin	cefalotin	Eli Lilly	antibiotic	infection
Hydergine	co-dergocrine mesylate	Sandoz	peripheral vasodilator	vasodilation
Indocid	indometacin	Merck	anti-inflammatory	arthritis
Inderal	propanolol	ICI	beta-blocker	hypertension
Brufen/Motrin	ibuprofen	Boots/Upjohn	anti-inflammatory	arthritis
Cefamezin	cefazolin	Erba	antibiotic	infection
Lasix	furosemide	Hoechst	diuretic	hypertension

		1985		
Brand name	Generic name	Company	Category	Indication
Tagamet	cimetidine	SKF	H_2 antagonist	peptic ulcer
Zantac	ranitidine	Glaxo	H_2 antagonist	peptic ulcer
Feldene	piroxicam	Pfizer	anti-inflammatory	arthritis
Tenormin	atenolol	ICI	beta-blocker	hypertension
Inderal	propanolol	ICI	beta-blocker	hypertension
Voltarol	diclofenac	Geigy	anti-inflammatory	arthritis
Naprosyn	naproxen	Syntex	anti-inflammatory	arthritis
Valium	diazepam	Roche	anxiolytic	anxiety
Amoxil	amoxicillin	Beecham	antibiotic	infection
Aldomet	methyldopa	Merck	hypotensive	hypertension

[a] Source: 1977 — Ciba Geigy, *Facts and Issues.*
              1985 — *SCRIP Yearbook*, 1987, p. 24-29.

countries (France, Federal Republic of Germany, Italy, Spain, and the United Kingdom) also shows interesting differences: the number of prescriptions for tranquillizers and hypnotics ranged from 0.2 per person per year in Spain to 0.7 in France and the Federal Republic of Germany; for non-steroid antirheumatics, from 0.31 in the Federal Republic of Germany to 0.7 in Italy; and for antibiotics from 0.16 in France to 0.68 in Spain (*18*). These differences can certainly not be explained by differences in morbidity. They can be more easily explained by irrational use of antibiotics or, in the case of tranquillizers and hypnotics, cultural differences.

Antibiotics account for a substantial proportion of the total drug budget in many countries and are often the largest single group of drugs purchased in developing countries. The consumption of antibiotics varies widely among countries. For example, Japan has a much higher consumption of cephalosporins than other countries and is the only country where cephalosporins are the most widely sold antibiotics; broad-spectrum antibiotics are the most common antibiotics in Mexico, Panama, and Spain; and tetracyclines are often prescribed in India, Norway, and Sweden (19).

There are many examples of the inappropriate use of antibiotics (20), but only limited data on the situation in developing countries. Much of the current information is anecdotal. In one study in Africa 50% of outpatients received at least one antibiotic (21). In a study in hospitals in Bangladesh, 57% of patients in the medical, surgical, and paediatric units received antibiotics, and only 50% of the prescriptions were considered to be appropriate (22). In Panama in 1979, a review of 266 anti-infective therapies in 339 hospitalized paediatric patients revealed that antibiotics were not used correctly in 210 cases (78.9%) (23). In a sample of 100 cases from a hospital in China, in only 59% was the use of antibiotics considered to be properly indicated (24).

Antibiotics are clearly not the only class of drugs to be misused. The volume of sales of certain drugs far exceeds the incidence of the disease they are supposed to treat. Cimetidine has proved beneficial in treating people with duodenal ulcers, but physicians have also been using it to treat a wide range of other conditions. In a study in Canada the authors found that "physicians prescribe cimetidine for diverse purposes most of which have not been validated" (25). In Brazil in 1986, over 500 million tranquillizers were consumed, an amount which, according to the Brazilian mental health specialists, far exceeds the real need (26). Many other examples (12) could be cited to show that, in both developed and developing countries, prescribing practices do not meet established scientific criteria and that, in spite of the many efforts, the situation has not improved during the last ten years as much as could have been expected (see Part II).

The consequences of this state of affairs are many: waste of public and private money, increase in iatrogenic diseases, etc. In the field of antibiotic use, resistance to newer antibacterials such as gentamicin or trimethoprim has been steadily increasing. Trimethoprim resistance is particularly important because there is no oral agent that is as effective or as cheap to replace it. The higher levels of resistance tend to be found in developing countries (27).

In addition to irrational prescription practices, patient non-compliance is nowadays considered to be a major problem in the health services of both developed and developing countries. A recent review of the literature suggests that the compliance rate for all treatments is approximately 50% and decreases with time (28). Another analysis showed that between 30% and 75% of patients do not take all the drugs prescribed, do not take them in the prescribed dosage, or use them wrongly; and that 40% of the mistakes could be harmful.[1] The low compliance rate for effective remedies results in the failure of curative or preventive treatment and may lead to extra expense for the patient and to the development of resistant strains.

Self-medication is another aspect of drug use and presents different features in developed and developing countries. In the developed countries ethical drugs cannot be purchased freely by consumers but must be prescribed by a physician. Self-medication concerns over-the-counter drugs, which are aimed at curing a vast array of aches, pains, discomfort and benign illnesses. In a number of developing countries, however, many ethical drugs are dispensed over the counter without medical supervision. In this case self-medication provides a lower-cost alternative for people who cannot afford to pay medical practitioners, and obviates long periods of waiting in overburdened health services (29). It is often the first response to illness among lower-income people. While most developing countries require pharmacies to employ at least one licensed pharmacist, he or she is not necessarily required to be present all the time; untrained assistant pharmacists, clerks, etc., are often responsible for dealing with patients, and their limited knowledge about drugs affects the choice of the product and the quantity and quality of information transmitted to the patient. Even when pharmacy personnel are well trained, their access to objective and accurate drug information is limited, and the economic incentive to sell the most expensive brands often influences their dispensing practices, thus extending the irrational use of drugs. Illegal purveyors of drugs (sellers in the markets, non-licensed providers of injections, etc.) are also common in developing countries and, along with some indigenous practitioners, a further source of irrational and potentially dangerous drug use. Traditional healers are increasingly incorporating modern drugs, including antibiotics, in their therapies. There is much anecdotal evidence of undesirable features in such self-medication — inappropriate purchasing of drugs for particular conditions, unfounded expectations — but few studies have quantified their extent.

In conclusion, it appears that the tremendously unequal distribution of drug consumption between developed and developing countries continues and that the gap, far from decreasing, is likely to widen. In developing countries, although per capita drug consumption at current prices was higher in 1985 than in 1976 (US$ 5.4 against US$ 3.4), the situation in constant prices has deteriorated in many countries, so that people spent less on drugs in 1985 than they did in 1976. Not only is the amount of money spent on drugs of concern (it is probably too high in developed countries and certainly too low in developing ones), drug consumption patterns and the use of drugs are

---

[1] HUYGUE, B. *La consommation et le mauvais usage des médicaments en Belgique 1970-1980.* Paper presented at a Colloquium of the Association des Epidémiologistes de Langue française (ADELF), Geneva, 1981.

also far from being rational. Allopathic drugs are being absorbed into diverse systems of health care but are often not used as they should be. However, all these indicators can only give a broad indication of the overall situation. Many developing countries, as will be described in Part II, have made good use of their scarce resources and, through rationalization of the drug sector, have been able to provide their population with a greater amout of essential drugs for the same money, and many developed countries have implemented cost containment measures and taken action to improve drug use.

Chapter 3

Drug supply

This chapter describes drug production and trade throughout the world and looks at the structure and dynamics of the pharmaceutical industry at the global level.

Drug production

Data on the production of pharmaceutical products are not available for a large number of countries, but it has been estimated that world pharmaceutical production has increased from US$ 29.6 billion (*30*) in 1973 to US$ 83.5 billion in 1980 and US$ 95.6 billion in 1985,[1] at current prices. The proportion produced in developing countries was 10.5% in 1973 and 11.5% in 1980; the objective of the Lima Declaration, that 25% of production should come from the Third World by the end of the century, is thus far from being achieved.

In both the developed and developing world, production capacity is highly concentrated in a few countries. In 1980, more than 90% of production took place in seven developed countries: the United States (30%), Japan (24%), the Federal Republic of Germany (13%), France (9%), the United Kingdom (6.4%), Italy (6%), and Switzerland (4%) (*31*).

Argentina, Brazil, Egypt, India, Mexico, and the Republic of Korea produce two-thirds of the output of developing countries. On average, in 1980 Latin American countries produced about 75% of their requirements for finished products, while Asian countries (excluding China) produced 60%. In Africa, most countries still depend very heavily on imports of finished products (*9*).

National estimates of production are of limited value. Many developing countries have a substantial drug industry, but it is largely made up of the local affiliates of foreign companies, the production of active ingredients and the development of new products taking place elsewhere.

---

[1] Estimates of UNIDO secretariat.

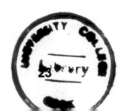

Trade[1]

Because of the wide range of needs for drugs throughout the world, and the concentration of production in industrialized countries, drugs are the subject of extensive international trade. In 1984, for example, total world imports represented US$ 8.9 billion.

International trade in drugs is carried out in two different forms: (1) as a raw material, shipped either in the form of chemical components or in bulk; and (2) as a finished product. The latter, at the world level, represents less than 60% of international trade in pharmaceutical products. Within the framework of the present survey, however, international trade in finished products[2] only will be studied.

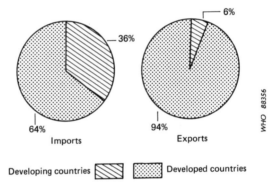

Fig. 4
Imports and exports of drugs in developed and developing countries, 1984.

---

[1] This discussion is limited to developed market economies.

[2] The Standard International Trade Classification (SITC) of the United Nations distinguishes between trade in medicaments (SITC 541.7) and overall trade in medicinal and pharmaceutical products (SITC 541), the latter including vitamins and provitamins, antibiotics (not included as medicaments), vegetable alkaloids, hormones, glycosides, and certain other pharmaceutical goods.

World import and export of medicaments and pharmaceuticals in 1984 was as follows (in billions of US$)

	Imports	Exports
Medicaments	8.974	8.560
Pharmaceuticals	15.769	14.716
Percentage	56.9	58.2

Source: *International trade statistics yearbook, 1984.* New York, United Nations, 1986.

For more details concerning the classification see *Standard international trade classification, revision 2.* New York, United Nations, 1975.

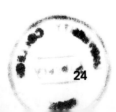

Almost all drug exports (94%) come from developed countries, and 64% of all imports are into developed countries. In other words, in most of international trade in drugs, developing countries play only a marginal role (Fig. 4).

Even though international trade in drugs with developing countries is marginal, imports of drugs are an essential element of the drug supply of these countries, drugs imported as finished products (medicaments) representing more than 20% of the total consumption. If all pharmaceutical imports are taken into account, the proportion reaches 41% (Table 11), a figure that underlines the heavy dependence of developing countries on foreign supplies of drugs.

Table 11.   Imports of drugs and pharmaceuticals and drug consumption in developed and developing countries, 1984 (billions of US$)[a]

	Total	Developing countries	Developed countries
Drug consumption	74.2	15.1	59.1
Imports of medicaments	8.9 (12%)[b]	3.2 (21.2%)	5.7 (9.6%)
Imports of pharmaceuticals	15.3 (20.6%)	6.2 (41.0%)	9.1 (15.4%)

[a] Source: *International trade statistics yearbook, 1984.* New York, United Nations, 1986.

[b] Figures in parentheses give percentage of total consumption.

In recent years financial constraints on the foreign supply of drugs have been particularly marked. As may be seen from Fig. 5, after the second oil price shock in 1979, the ensuing slower economic growth, and the debt

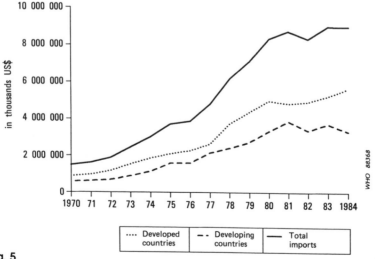

Fig. 5
Evolution of world drug imports.

crisis a few years later, the increase in imports of drugs slowed down throughout the world and in particular in developing countries. Whereas between 1970 and 1980 the average annual growth rate in drug imports was 18.9%, between 1980 and 1984 it decreased to 1.9%. In developing countries the slowdown was even more dramatic, from 20.8% between 1970 and 1980 to −1.3% between 1980 and 1984. Lower inflation rates and a less dynamic overall international trade situation only partly explain this slowdown, the major reason, particularly for developing countries, being fewer financial resources.

Despite this slowdown, the structure of international trade in drugs has not changed drastically. European countries remained in 1984, as in 1970, the largest drug importers (42% of world drug imports) and the largest drug exporters (77.5% of world drug exports) (Table 12).

Table 12. **Distribution of drug imports and exports by region in 1970 and 1984**[a]

	Imports (%)		Exports (%)	
	1970	1984	1970	1984
Africa	14.2	10.2	0.2	0.2
Latin America	8.5	6.5	2.0	1.7
Asia	16.6	18.9	3.2	3.6
Developing countries	39.3	35.6	5.4	5.5
European countries	44.1	42.4	79.1	77.5
North America	2.2	10.9	12.2	14.0
Japan	8.7	7.5	1.9	0.9
Other developed countries	5.7	3.6	1.4	2.1
Developed countries	60.7	64.4	94.6	94.5

[a] Source: *International trade statistics yearbook, 1984*. New York, United Nations, 1986.

This predominance may be partly explained by the large amount of drugs exchanged within Europe and the formal links that exist between several European countries and developing countries; 50.9% of European exports go to other European countries, 12.7% to Africa, and 19.6% to Asia (Table 13).

The concentration of imports originating mainly from Europe is another important issue for developing countries. Most of the drugs imported into Africa come from Europe (96%), as well as 58.4% of those imported into Asia. This concentration increases dependence on limited sources of supply

Table 13. Distribution of European imports and exports of drugs, 1984[a]

	Europe	Africa	Latin America	North America	Asia[b]	Other
Imports (%)	93.0	0.1	0.1	5.2	0.8	0.8
Exports (%)	50.9	12.7	3.4	5.1	19.6	8.3

[a] Source: United Nations Comtrade data bank, as of August 1987.
[b] Including Japan.

and creates trade flows that are often difficult to change (Table 14). Only in Latin America is there evidence of some trade between developing countries; 31.6% of drugs imported into Latin American countries come from another Latin American country (Table 14).

Table 14. Sources of drug imports to African, Asian, and Latin American countries, 1984[a]

	Europe	Africa	Latin America	North America	Asia[b]	Other
Africa	96.0	0.7	0.1	2.4	0.5	0.3
Latin America	49.3	–	31.6	13.0	1.0	5.1
Asia[b]	58.4	–	0.2	22.6	16.6	2.2

[a] Source: United Nations Comtrade data bank, as of August 1987.
[b] Including Japan.

Drug suppliers

Drug producers can be divided into three broad categories: (1) producers in developing countries; (2) generic producers in the developed world; and (3) large research and development-oriented firms that market their drugs primarily under brand names. Most production, trade, and sales of drugs are in the hands of these firms, which, with very few exceptions, are multinational corporations with headquarters in developed countries.

Local producers in developing countries

Developing countries range from those with total dependence on imported finished products to those that manufacture medicinal chemicals and active ingredients. Each level of development has a distinctive set of constraints (see Part II).

Transnational corporations generally play a dominant role, their share of the market ranging from 30% in Egypt, 50% in Argentina, 70% in India, 78% in Brazil, and 90% in Ecuador to nearly 100% in many African countries (6). Subsidiaries of the major pharmaceutical companies may or may not have national capital participation, depending on the law of the country. They generally produce pharmaceuticals developed by the parent firms and buy the raw materials from the parent companies. In some cases, for reasons of taxation and profit, it is in the interest of the companies to sell the active ingredients to the subsidiary at a high price, thus increasing the cost of production. This practice, called transfer pricing, has been well documented by the United Nations Centre on Transnational Corporations (9). The multinational companies function in the same way as in developed countries, through product and promotional rivalry.

A large number of domestically owned pharmaceutical firms, engaged mainly in formulation and packaging, compete for the remaining share of the market. These firms may be privately owned or state-owned and, because they are not able to carry out research and development, often market a wide range of drugs that are combination or duplicate products. National producers, because of their size and the need to employ hard currency for technology and raw materials, are very vulnerable to changes in the economy and in government policies.

To increase local ownership, many developing countries have been promoting joint ventures between foreign and national companies. A bilateral cooperation agreement usually includes a commitment by the new industry in the developing country to buy active ingredients, packing materials, or technology from its international partner. The international partner is committed to investing capital, transferring technology, training personnel, and selling raw materials to the new industry. Most developing countries in recent decades have developed an interest in the local production of drugs, as a way of improving their economy and decreasing their dependence. In many cases, however, there is a conflict between economic policy and health policy (see Part II).

Generic producers in developed countries

Generic drugs are unpatented drug products, including drugs whose patent has expired and those that have never been patented. The generic market is divided into two segments: branded generics, which are unpatented products sold under a brand name, and commodity generics, which are sold under a generic name and marketed by a wide variety of companies at low prices.

Since the mid-1970s, the trend in the pharmaceutical industry, particularly in the United States of America, has been towards expanding the generic industry. For some observers "the emergence of the US generics market should be considered a milestone event — perhaps a breakthrough in the evolution and transformation of the world pharmaceutical industry and, indeed, the entire pharmaceutical supply system" (32). Several factors have influenced this trend:

1. Many of the best-selling products in the market are losing their patent protection. Between 1975 and 1987, 56 major products lost patent coverage, and 64 others will lose it by 1989 (33). Only 21 of the top 100 prescription drugs in the USA in 1986 will still have patent protection in 1990 (34).

2. Increased cost-consciousness on the part of both governments and consumers in the public and private sector has led to the adoption of cost-containment measures in many countries.

3. The parallel importing practice within the European Economic Community, by which wholesalers buy branded products in a country where prices are low and sell them in another one, has stimulated the debate on generic drugs.

4. The influence of the WHO Action Programme on Essential Drugs and of the concepts underlying it is growing.

5. The Drug Price Competition and Patent Restoration Act, also called the Waxman–Hatch Act (1984), has been the single most effective factor in opening up the generic market in the United States. This Act can be viewed as a compromise between the research-based industries and the generic producers, its aim being to stimulate price competition while at the same time rewarding innovation. It supersedes the 1962 Act, which required generic versions of drugs to undergo clinical trials duplicating the safety and efficacy data collected by the inventors. The 1984 Act requires the applicant for a licence to demonstrate to the Food and Drug Administration that the product is equivalent to the original one in terms of bioavailability and effects. It also grants an extension of the period of market exclusivity to the discoverers of new drugs by allowing them to recapture some of the years that the drug is under review by the Food and Drug Administration.

6. The development of state substitution laws in the USA has stimulated the demand for generics. These laws vary greatly in scope but allow pharmacists to substitute generic products for branded ones. In most states, however, physicians may refuse substitution.

Among the developed countries the USA has the largest generic market: 25% of the total in 1985 (Table 15). This market, which was estimated as 20% of the total in 1978, will, according to a number of industrial analysts, grow to 35% by 1990 (35). The percentage of prescriptions written in generic terms in the United States increased steadily from 9.2% in 1974 to 36% in 1987 (36).

Generic substitution (i.e., the percentage of prescriptions supplied as generics but written by brand) also increased from 26.4% in 1984 to 35.7%

Table 15. Percentage market shares of generics in certain countries, 1980–1985[a]

Country	1980	1981	1982	1983	1984	1985
France	n.a[b]	1.0	1.0	2.0	2.0	3.0
Federal Republic of Germany	1.5	1.5	2.5	3.0	4.0	5.0
United Kingdom	3.0	3.0	4.0	6.0	7.0	9.0
Italy	6.0	9.0	9.0	9.5	10.0	11.0
Japan	12.0	14.0	15.0	15.0	17.0	19.0
Canada	n.a[b]	14.1	17.5	18.5	19.9	21.3
USA	21.0	21.0	22.0	22.0	24.0	25.0

[a] Source: *Pharmaceutical executive*, quoted in *Scrip Yearbook*, 1987, p. 45.

[b] Data not available.

in 1985. Of a sample of 10 drugs, 8 were substituted by generics in about 30% of cases in 1985 and the other 2 in more than 50% (*37*).

In other developed countries the generic market is growing at a slower pace, the substitution of commodity generics encountering resistance from various groups. In France one company introduced several generic products in 1980. However, after strong protests from the National Pharmacists' Association, the marketing of these drugs to retail pharmacists was suspended; sales to hospitals continued. As in many other European countries, retail pharmaceutical margins in France are fixed by law as a percentage of the price to the public; there is therefore no economic incentive for a pharmacist to promote lower-priced generic drugs. This situation is a major barrier to growth of the generic market in Europe (*33*). Nevertheless, in many cases generic companies are increasing their market share. In the Federal Republic of Germany, for example, in the mono-preparations market, manufacturers of generic drugs achieved a market share of 13% in terms of value in 1985 (*38*).

The companies involved in the manufacture and marketing of generic drugs are heterogeneous in terms of size, scope of activities, and resources. Both generic companies and research and development companies are engaged in the supply of generic drugs. There are 600 generic pharmaceutical manufacturers in the United States (*31*), ranging from big firms like the Rugby Group (one of the leaders in the market with estimated sales of US$ 200 million in 1984) to very small firms with fewer than 10 salaried employees and US$ 20 million sales per year (*35*). Many research and development companies market *de facto* branded generics, since they continue to sell their products after the expiry of the patent. Roche, for example, continues to market branded Librium in the face of multisource competition from both branded and commodity generics (*33*). Other companies made the decision to enter the commodity generic market either under their own name with a specific product line (Lederle) or by acquiring generic companies (Ciba-Geigy).

No one company has a majority share of the commodity generic market, the total sales of the ten leaders in 1984 in the USA accounting for less than 7% of the total generic market there (35).

At the international level the success of the generics policy in the United States will certainly have important repercussions. For many years the generics issue has been the subject of numerous debates. Some developing countries have tried to implement generics policies, and many attempts have failed. The present situation in the United States may stimulate new developments and new initiatives around the world.

Among other consequences of the introduction of generic competitors is increased competition, mainly relating to price. A recent report of the Federal Trade Commission in the USA estimated that, in 1984, generic drugs saved consumers approximately US$ 236 million in the United States (39). In 1985 in the same country, the average price of the generic products was US$ 6.62, as compared with US$ 12.78 for brand-name products (40). Another study showed that, for each of 51 matched drugs, the generic product was always cheaper. The saving achieved in buying the generic product ranged from 7.5% for flurazepam to 61.8% for diphenhydramine and 80.1% for meclozine. The average saving for the top 20 products was 49.2% (41). In the Netherlands in 1987 generics were 15% cheaper than brand-name products (26).

Another result of generic competition is an increased demand by consumers for proof, before they agree to pay higher prices for a drug, that the added benefit justifies the cost. Yet another result is changes in the strategies of research and development-based companies in a way that is not yet very clear, but is probably in the direction of their becoming more customer-oriented than doctor-oriented, and focused on innovative products. Growth opportunities are also being afforded to companies specializing in the supply of raw materials to the large pharmaceutical companies. In the United States, competition has increased among pharmaceutical chemical manufacturers.

Research-based pharmaceutical companies

Although the pharmaceutical industry comprises 10 000 companies worldwide, no more than 100 companies, the large research and development-oriented firms, have a significant share of the international market, and over the years they have tended to remain the market leaders, only their rank shifting, as shown in Table 16. In 1985 these firms supplied 80% of

Table 16.   World's fifteen largest pharmaceutical companies by sales, 1977–1985[a]

	Country	1977	1980	1981	1982	1983	1984	1985
Hoechst	FRG	1	1	1	1	1	3	3
Merck & Co.	USA	2	3	3	3	3	1	1
Bayer	FRG	3	2	2	2	2	4	5
Ciba-Geigy	SWI	4	4	4	5	5	5	4
Hoffmann La Roche	SWI	5	6	7	8	10	11	15
American Home Products	USA	6	5	6	4	4	2	2
Warner Lambert	USA	7	9	11	14	13	14	7
Pfizer	USA	8	8	5	6	6	6	6
Sandoz	SWI	9	7	8	9	12	12	14
Eli Lilly	USA	10	11	9	7	7	8	9
Upjohn	USA	11	–	12	–	14	13	13
Boehringer Ingelheim	FRG	12	13	15	15	–	–	–
Squibb	USA	13	15	14	–	–	–	–
Bristol Myers	USA	14	12	10	10	9	9	10
Takeda	JAP	15	10	–	13	15	15	–
Smith Kline	USA	–	14	13	11	11	10	12
Glaxo	UK	–	–	–	–	–	–	11
Abbott	USA	–	–	–	12	8	7	8

[a] Sources:
1977 – *Transnational corporations and the pharmaceutical industry*, New York, UNCTC, 1979;
1980 – *SCRIP* No. 653/4, 21 and 24 December 1981;
1981 – *SCRIP* No. 755, 20 and 22 December 1982;
1982 – *SCRIP* No. 857 and 858, 21 and 26 December 1983;
1983 – *SCRIP* No. 959, 19 December 1984;
1984 – *SCRIP* No. 1063/4, 25 December 1985;
1985 – *SCRIP* No. 1166/7, 25 December 1986 and 1 January 1987.

world shipments of pharmaceutical products, the top 50 accounting for over two-thirds of this total, the first 25 for about a half (*41*).

While these figures show that the drug industry is not a monopoly, it should be borne in mind that the pharmaceutical market is divided into a number of separate therapeutic markets. Thus, in the world market for anti-ulcer/antacid drugs, one company accounts for 28% of total sales and five companies for 57.7%. In the market for anti-asthmatic drugs, the proportion is 18.8% for the top company and 48% for the top five (*37*). Thus, the concentration within specific therapeutic markets is much higher and determines the exact nature of the competition.

All the top companies are transnational corporations. They sell their products in foreign markets, their involvement outside their home markets depending to a large extent on the size of their national market and the number of major pharmaceutical companies in their home market. Thus

European firms are the most internationalized; between 30% (France) and 90% (Switzerland) of their sales are outside their home markets (43).

There has been a general increase in the level of foreign sales among the top companies. In 1981 about 54% of the sales of the top 30 companies were in foreign markets, the corresponding figure in 1984 being 73%. Companies ranked below 130 are mainly oriented to the domestic market, their foreign sales representing less than 10% of their total sales (43).

Corporations based in the United States of America are clearly the world leaders today; seven were among the top ten companies in 1985 and 15 among the top 30 (43). This represents a marked change since 1974, an increased role being played by American companies. This can be explained partly by the increased share of the American market in the world market (Table 2) but also by the internationalization of United States companies. Their subsidiaries in other countries accounted for 20% of total sales of United States firms in 1960, 30% in 1972, 42% in 1979, and about 50% more recently (31). These facts explain the growing interest of the US pharmaceutical industry in the drug situation throughout the world.

Several special features have for many years characterized the pharmaceutical industry. First, its products are highly patented. Second, price has not traditionally been a significant factor in determining the demand for pharmaceutical products. Third, the success of individual companies stems primarily from innovation (i.e., success in introducing new drugs) and promotion strategies.

For an understanding of the world drug situation and the future outlook, it is useful to review briefly the evolution of the industry and the key changes that have taken place in recent years. Historically, changes in the industry have been rather slow. Today, according to many observers, a series of dynamic trends in numerous areas will probably have a major impact on the pharmaceutical industry and thus on the world drug situation.

For many years prior to 1940 the industry was essentially a production-oriented manufacturer of commodity products, engaged primarily in the manufacture and marketing of products that had been available for many years. Between 1905 and 1935, for example, an average of six new drugs were added each year to the United States Pharmacopeia. The industry supplied the active ingredient to retail pharmacists, who produced the final compound in finished dosage form. The cost of goods represented between 65% and 70% of total sales; and drug technology was fixed, so that expenditure on research and development was fairly low (33). Advertising focused on the consumer, as no distinction was made between ethical and over-the-counter drugs.

Outstanding scientific and technological advances during the 1940s and 1950s resulted in the development of a whole new range of drugs. With this wave of "wonder drugs" the pharmaceutical companies became vertically integrated, combining production of raw materials, drug research and manufacture, and marketing. Expenditure on research and development increased to about 8% of total sales, the cost of goods being only 25–30% of total sales. Innovation became the critical factor for the survival of any company. There has been a continuous effort to introduce into the market newer substitutes that could displace older drugs and thus maintain or increase the market share. During the 1950s and 1960s an average of 444 products were placed on the market each year, only 10% being new chemical entities (33). As a consequence of this proliferation of products the industry developed a marketing strategy based on heavy promotion among physicians in order to create brand loyalty and achieve high prices for products, especially when first introduced on the market. The industry shifted from being a non-prescription to primarily a prescription drug industry with the physician as the principal target for promotion. The competition pattern set up was thus based on product differentiation, patents, and brand names.

The introduction of some of the new drugs was accompanied by major disasters, e.g., that associated with the use of thalidomide. Following these tragedies, government regulation increased in most countries during the 1960s.

Since the 1960s, the pharmaceutical industry has preserved the same characteristics and has acquired a new one: internationalization. The drug companies have expanded into new markets, extending their operations throughout the world to ensure that their products are sold as widely as possible.

Research and development

Research and development remain the principal mechanisms whereby society is supplied with new drugs to prevent, control, and cure disease. They are also extremely important for pharmaceutical firms in maintaining growth and competitive advantage; investment in research and development has to generate products that can be sold in large markets at reasonable profit. Accordingly, economic and social concerns are often in conflict.

The leading companies on the world market (see Table 16) are also the top companies with regard to the number of products under development (Table 17). Together France, the Federal Republic of Germany, Italy, Japan,

Switzerland, the United Kingdom, and the United States of America in 1982 accounted for three-quarters of the pharmaceutical industry's expenditure on the search for new medicines — an estimated US$ 5.5 billion (44). In 1984 the expenditure was estimated to be US$ 6.5 billion (35). The expenditure for the pharmaceutical industry in the USA, as shown in Table 18, has increased substantially during the past two decades (although since the 1960s it has remained as a more or less constant percentage of pharmaceutical sales).

Table 17. Top research-based companies, according to number of entities introduced, 1961–1985[a]

Company/concern	Country	No. of entities
Hoechst	Federal Republic of Germany	67
Rhône-Poulenc	France	61
Johnson & Johnson	USA	50
Sanofi	France	49
Sandoz	Switzerland	44
Bayer	Federal Republic of Germany	42
Boehringer Ingelheim	Federal Republic of Germany	41
Hoffmann La Roche	Switzerland	40
Ciba-Geigy	Switzerland	38
Merck & Co.	USA	30
Pfizer	USA	29
Upjohn	USA	28
Montedison	Italy	27
Lilly	USA	26
Warner Lambert	USA	26
L'Oréal	France	23
Schering AG	Federal Republic of Germany	23
Dow	USA	22
Glaxo	United Kingdom	22
Syntex	USA	22
Takeda	Japan	21
Beecham	United Kingdom	19
Bristol	USA	19
Merck	Federal Republic of Germany	19

[a] Source: REIS-ARNDT, E. A quarter of a century of pharmaceutical research. *Drugs made in Germany*. 30: 105–112 (1987).

Both the cost of research and the time required to transfer a drug from the laboratory to the market have increased in the last 15 years. In 1963 in the United Kingdom, according to industry analysts, it took about three years and £2–3 million to develop and market a new drug; now it is estimated that it takes 7–10 years and £50 million. In the Federal Republic of

Table 18.   Global research and development expenditure as compared with sales for the pharmaceutical industry in the USA[a]

Year	Global sales[b]	Global research and development[b]	Research and development as % of sales
1951	1 350	50	3.70
1952	1 400	63	4.50
1953	1 450	67	4.62
1954	1 500	78	5.20
1955	1 650	91	5.52
1956	1 900	105	5.53
1957	2 200	127	5.77
1958	2 400	170	7.08
1959	2 500	197	7.88
1960	2 600	212	8.15
1961	2 685	238	8.86
1962	2 932	251	8.56
1963	3 152	282	8.95
1964	3 405	298	8.75
1965	3 841	351	9.14
1966	4 256	402	9.45
1967	4 707	448	9.52
1968	5 280	485	9.19
1969	5 832	549	9.41
1970	6 442	619	9.61
1971	7 020	684	9.74
1972	7 827	726	9.28
1973	8 755	825	9.42
1974	10 120	942	9.31
1975	11 543	1 062	9.20
1976	12 832	1 164	9.07
1977	13 896	1 276	9.18
1978	16 040	1 404	8.75
1979	18 422	1 627	8.83
1980	21 460	1 860	8.67
1981	22 378	2 211	9.88
1982	24 466	2 641	10.80
1983	26 254	3 063	11.67
1984	28 496	3 531	12.39
1985	31 562	3 956	12.53

[a] Source: *Annual survey*, Washington, DC, Pharmaceutical Manufacturers Association.

[b] Figures are in millions of US dollars and include products for both human and veterinary use.

Germany, the average duration of research and development on new substances increased from 2.3 years for research and 5 years for development in 1964 to 9 and 13 years in 1981, with a cost in 1981 of between DM 150 and 300 million (US$ 57–114 million) (*44*).

In the United States development time increased from 2 to 7–10 years and cost from US$ 54 million in 1976 to US$ 75–100 million in 1985.[1] A new study funded by the United States Pharmaceutical Manufacturers Association suggests that in 1986, the cost of developing a new chemical entity had risen to US$ 125 million (US$ 65 million out-of-pocket expenditure and US$ 60 million as opportunity cost) (45). These figures are averages and cover the failures as well as the successes. Some industry analysts consider that much of the cost must relate to research and development projects that do not succeed. The actual cost of developing a new chemical entity must therefore be far less (46).

The productivity of research and development expenditure can be gauged by the number of new chemical entities appearing on the market. A recent survey revealed that 1787 products were introduced into the world pharmaceutical market over the period 1961–85 and that the annual total declined from an average of 85 per year in 1961–71 to 55 per year over the period 1976–85. The seven countries mentioned earlier continued to be the major source of new pharmaceutical preparations; in 1961 they accounted for 88% of new chemical entities, and for 95% in 1985. During the period 1961–85 most of the new compounds were developed in the USA, followed by France, the Federal Republic of Germany, and Japan. In recent years Japan has taken second place, with 61 new compounds in the last five years compared with 69 in the United States. During the period 1961–85 Eastern Europe developed 113 drugs (14).

A number of factors in recent years have contributed to a lower output of new chemical entities and to an increase in the cost of making new drugs available on the market. They include reduced opportunities for innovation, requirement for more costly methods for detecting toxicological problems, and more stringent regulation. Regulation affects profitability by increasing the time and cost involved in placing a drug on the market. It could also affect the decision to take on certain minor research projects. No one, however, denies that regulation is an important element in protecting consumers from toxic and/or ineffective drugs.

The decline has been mainly in the total number of drugs introduced annually, and not the number of new chemical entities (Fig. 6). In the United States of America in 1950 the total number of new products was 326; of these 198 were new combination products, 100 were duplicate single products, and 28 were new chemical entities; in 1983 the total number of new products was 123, of which 41 were combination drugs, 60 were duplicate single drugs, and 22 were new chemical entities. Therefore, newly

---

[1] According to some sources, this figure suggests that roughly half of the industry's research and development expenditure goes to development of new chemical entities. The other half is spent on other research and development activities (extensions of current products, regulatory defence of current products, etc.) (35).

synthesized drugs represented 9% of all new products in 1950, and 18% in 1983. The decline in the introduction of new drugs seems to have been confined largely to drugs of secondary importance.

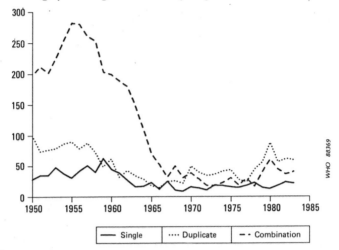

Fig. 6
Introduction of new products in the United States of America, 1950–83.

Sources: FULDA, T.R. *Prescription drug data summary 1974.* Washington, DC, Office of Research and Statistics, 1976 (HEW Publication No. (SSA) 76-11928); DE HAEN, P. *Ten-year new product survey, 1950-1960; Non-proprietary name index,* Vol. VI, New York, Paul de Haen Inc.; *De Haen new product survey. Pharmaceutical specialities introduced in the United States, 1974-1983,* New York, Paul de Haen Inc., 1984.

During the past decade the internationalization of research and development has increased. American companies, which in 1976 spent 8% of their research and development budget abroad, spent more than 20% outside the United States at the beginning of the 1980s. Swiss companies spent nearly 40% outside their home country, and the other European companies 10–20%. The most important reason for using foreign research facilities is the desire to exploit the scientific resources of another country. Thus, very few investments are made in developing countries and, according to a study carried out by Pharma Information (*1*), those few are often the result of political pressure.

Although research and development are still concentrated in developed countries, there are some examples of developing countries investing in this area. China has given top priority to biotechnology in its science and technology development programme (*48*), while Brazil is investing in a new National Centre for Biotechnology Research linked to the National University of Campinas (*49*).

Data on the number of new chemical entities, however, do not give any indication of the quality or relevance of the research. The Food and Drug Administration in the United States and Barral (*47*) in France have developed a classification that takes into account the therapeutic relevance

of the drugs developed and marketed. Barral defines the following
categories according to the structure of the compound and the therapeutic
improvement achieved:

A. new structure; therapeutic improvement;

B. well known structure; therapeutic improvement;

C. new structure; no therapeutic improvement;

D. well known structure; no therapeutic improvement.

Analysing the 508 new chemical entities marketed during the period
1975–84, Barral found the distribution by group shown in Table 19.

Table 19. Distribution of new drugs according to Barral's classification[a]

Category	No. of drugs	%
A	35	6.9
B	115	22.6
C	75	14.8
D	283	55.7
Total	508	100.0

[a] Source: BARRAL, E. *Prospective et santé*, No. 36, Winter 1985-86, p. 90.

Of the 508 new chemical entities, 398 were not new structures, which
means that research was carried out on existing molecules to find new
therapeutic applications or improvements. Improvements were obtained
for 115 of them. Of the 110 new structures, 75 revealed no therapeutic
advantages over existing products.

Of the 508 products, 52 were antibiotics (23 of which were cephalosporins),
31 were anti-cancer products (mainly in category B), 85 were for cardiovascular disease, 60 for central nervous system disorders (most of the
anxiolytics being benzodiazepines), 11 were anti-ulcer drugs, and 56 were
anti-inflammatory drugs (47, 50). Analysis of the products in different stages
of development each year shows the same trends; since 1980 the
therapeutic category with the greatest number of products in research and
development has been that of neurological drugs (Table 20). However, with
the spread of acquired immunodeficiency syndrome, it is likely that many
companies will step up research on anti-viral products.

The main factors that influence research priorities are, according to the
pharmaceutical industry: (1) the strength of the market signals being
received and (2) technical feasibility and the need to achieve a balance
between generating products that can contribute to better health and
ensuring a continuing flow of income (51).

Table 20. Compounds under research and development by therapeutic class, 1981–1986[a, b]

	1981	1982	1983	1984	1985	1986
Dietetic	250	294	332	359	435	480
Blood and clotting	196	232	271	310	387	451
Cardiovascular	469	459	528	594	816	962
Dermatological	81	82	94	117	160	217
Gynaecological/urological (including sex hormones)	104	113	131	122	153	173
Hormones excluding sex hormones	124	135	140	161	187	204
Anti-infective drugs	514	513	583	611	813	955
Anti-cancer drugs	378	451	522	597	818	909
Musculoskeletal	221	236	264	270	340	422
Neurological	582	574	650	699	851	967
Against parasites	46	53	55	58	76	87
Respiratory	166	173	196	227	290	352

[a] Source: see footnote a, Table 16.

[b] Because many products have more than one activity and are repeated during the different years, the total in the table far exceeds Barral's total.

Although a number of products developed during the last ten years have a secondary indication for the treatment of tropical diseases, few new drugs have been developed primarily for use against such diseases: these include, for example, mefloquine, praziquantel, oxamniquine, benznidazole, secnidazole and ivermectin (47). However, some promising drugs are still under development: artemisinine and halofantrine for malaria and eflornithine for African trypanosomiasis. Advances in biotechnology and related areas also hold out the promise of new cost-effective techniques of immunization against diseases such as malaria, viral hepatitis B, leprosy, rotavirus infections, etc. The annual expenditure on research and development by the pharmaceutical industry in tropical medicine is not known, but a report by the Office of Health Economics reveals that the six European companies most actively involved in this kind of research spent US$ 30 million in 1976–77 (direct costs and overheads), US$ 33 million in 1979–80, and US$ 40 million in 1982–83 (52). Taking into account the world sales of these six companies and assuming that 10% of sales revenue was devoted to research and development, tropical disease research and development do not account for more than 4% of the total research investment of these firms. This means that, as a whole, the industry is probably spending much less than 4% of its research budget in this area. Investment is therefore urgently needed, but as the pharmaceutical industry has explained, it seems unrealistic to expect companies to fund research with few prospects of recovering their costs. These is thus a need for new schemes, such as the UNDP/World Bank/WHO Special Programme for Research and Training in Tropical Diseases.

In the future research and development are likely to continue to become more complex, time-consuming, and costly. A consequence will be the emergence of three types of firm, one producing mainly generic products and two being engaged in research and development (*53*). The difference between these two would be in the amount of investment in research and development; the high cost of research and development will mean that only a dozen or so companies will be able to afford it and they will focus more and more on a selected range of therapeutic entities and on truly innovative new agents with a clear medical need, a large market, and considerable profit potential. As shown in Barral's study (*47*), the degree of commercial success is directly proportional to the level of innovation; the rate of success for category A products was 80%, for B products 59%, for C products 37%, and for D products 31%. Apparently many companies think they are able to produce innovative drugs, as illustrated by the fact that their research and development budgets have increased in recent years (*54*). Overall, the major companies since 1980 have increased their expenditure on research and development. According to *SCRIP* (*43*) the top ten spend more than 15% of their sales revenue on research and development, and the top 30 more than 12%. Greater emphasis is now being put on research efficiency.

Although some experts estimate that 75–85% of all the new chemical entities currently awaiting approval by the Food and Drug Administration belong to the imitative category (*35*), advances in the biological and biochemical sciences in recent years are likely to foster the development of major new therapeutic agents, more specifically the products of what some have called the "second pharmacological revolution". They include neuro-transmitters, mood-altering drugs, prostaglandins, and products to treat the health problems of the elderly (the fastest-growing population group in the major world markets) (*31*).

Many of the drugs of the future will also be products of recombinant DNA technology. Until now, genetic engineering has mainly offered ways of making and improving old products (e.g., human insulin), but new products are on the way, though their appearance on the market may take longer than expected.

Novel drug delivery systems and techniques for carrying agents to specific receptor sites will also be a new field for expansion and one of the responses of research and development firms to the threatening growth of the generic producers. The goal will be to replace current "peak and trough" dosing systems with ones that provide the medicinal effect when and where needed (*31*).

Patents and brand names

Once companies have invested in the research, development, and marketing of a drug, they expect to enjoy a period without competition in which they can recover their investment and make profits. Society acknowledges and promotes research by granting patents. There are two types of patent protection: product patent, which covers the substance itself, and process patent, which covers only the method of manufacture. The latter does not provide very strong protection for the innovator. Until the 1950s most countries relied only on process patents for pharmaceuticals (52). However, since then most developed countries have introduced product patents. The function of a patent is primarily to stimulate inventive activity by preventing a new product from being imitated during a legally sanctioned period (17 years from the date of issue in the United States of America, 20 years from the date of application for most European countries).

In developing countries, patent protection for pharmaceuticals has two aspects. On the one hand it can provide a favourable atmosphere for foreign investment, protect domestic innovation, foster foreign innovation in drugs that have their main markets in developing countries, and facilitate domestic licensing. On the other hand, according to a UNIDO report (30), patents have often been used to secure import monopolies (stopping the importation of cheaper products) and to prevent local manufacturers from producing similar products.

In the 1970s, many developing countries fought to abolish or at least revise the international patent system, but with little success. Nowadays, pressure from research-based pharmaceutical industry is mounting in favour of product protection in developing countries and extension of the patent term to 20 years and more in developed countries, the principal reason being to compensate for the time taken to complete the increasingly stringent tests and trials required by the authorities to establish safety and efficacy (55). In the USA, this pressure led to the 1984 Drug Price Competition and Patent Term Restoration Act, which extends by up to five years the time lost while new drugs are being evaluated for approval (56). In Japan it led to a proposed bill requesting a five-year extension of the patent term to 20 years (41), in Canada to legislation that would largely repeal compulsory licensing (36), in the Federal Republic of Germany to steps to prolong the commercial life of innovative products (41). The question is more complex than it appears at first. Some governments, mainly in the European Economic Community, doubt the validity of the industry's arguments. The key concern of these authorities is whether they are in fact "being asked to support, through patent term extension, either an inefficient system for developing new drugs or an industry which, for commercial reasons, is becoming increasingly restrictive in what it regards as economically viable new products. For companies with total sales well in excess of US$ 1 000 million a year, a new product with an international sales potential of less than US$ 200 million may well be classified as commercially uninteresting" (55). Patent term extension can compensate to some extent for lack of success in research and development.

In many developing countries steps are being taken to increase pharmaceutical products and process patent protection. Pressures are mounting from those concerned with patent protection and are giving rise to intensive discussion. Product patents were introduced in the Republic of Korea in mid-1987 (57). Mexico has developed a project for additions to and reforms of laws governing inventions and brand names by which process patents will be introduced and a product patent system developed over a period of ten years. Brazil and Colombia are being urged to introduce patent protection while Argentina is being persuaded to move to a product patent system (58). In mid-1986, at the first Latin American Pharmaceutical Industry Forum, one of the most significant topics of debate was the "growing threat posed to the region by industrialized countries seeking to obtain legislative changes to allow patent protection for drug products" (59). According to domestic companies, these changes would cripple the national industry.

In Asia, Indonesia (60), Thailand (61), and other countries are being submitted to the same pressures. In mid-1987 Thailand was urged to amend its patent legislation to include pharmaceuticals. The Thai domestic pharmaceutical industry was opposed to such a change on the grounds that prices of pharmaceutical products would rise if patent protection was introduced and that it did not promote the transfer of technology, as had been shown previously in other sectors of industry that came under the patent law.

Many developing countries still basically agree with the conclusion of the 1978 UNIDO report on the subject: "In a country with little industry, a case may be made for weakening the patent system to receive the benefits of cheap imports. In countries with developing pharmaceutical industry, there is a case for keeping the system with a number of safeguards so that its potentially restrictive effects on domestic development are minimized. In countries engaged in major research and development, the case is clear for a fairly strong patent system" (30, 62).

The product brand name system is a vital complement to the patent system. Brand names are a means of achieving product differentiation and may be effective when patents are not and when products lose their patents. One of the consequences of the brand name system is the large number of different names for the same drug: there are in the world about 100 000 brand-name drugs, and some drugs such as antibiotics, tranquillizers, and analgesics can be found in some countries under 200 brand names. This proliferation of products makes price competition difficult as the physician generally finds it easier to work with a few well promoted brands. The brand name system is therefore the foundation of the drug industry's extensive promotional activity, on which the industry spends more than 20% of its sales revenue. Drug promotion is meant to provide physicians with essential scientific information about a wide variety of new products. In addition to the educational purpose, however, a goal of the promotional programme is to gain and maintain market dominance for the industry's products through the creation of strong and lasting brand name preferences among both prescribing physicians and the public (63).

Drug promotion has always been a controversial issue and the subject of detailed investigations. In many surveys carried out during the 1970s important differences were observed in the ways drugs were promoted among physicians in developed and in developing countries. As a result of the increased pressure from consumer movements and governments, the International Federation of Pharmaceutical Manufacturers Association (IFPMA) developed a voluntary code of marketing practices in 1981, and WHO was asked to convene a meeting of experts in 1987 to develop ethical criteria for drug promotion. In 1984 a new survey was undertaken which found that many of the pharmaceutical firms were limiting their promotional claims in the Third World to those supported by scientific evidence and were more willing to disclose side-effects. There is, however, room for further improvement on the part of both multinational and domestic companies (64).

As it is in the interest of a specific drug company to promote its own drug, irrespective of its therapeutic value and its price, promotion can result in the use of inferior medicines or the overutilization of effective and costly drugs. In Canada, for example, a review of the national drug compendium revealed that 35.7% of the products are irrational combinations whose prescribing and use are to a large extent due to promotion (65). In the United States promotion is widely used in the battle of the research and development companies against generic competition, firstly in the form of aggressive advertising to physicians and pharmacists regarding the benefits of their products as compared with generics, and secondly in the form of promotion of a new look for older drugs (many companies are making major changes in the appearance of their branded products) so as to create brand loyalty among physicians and patients (66). Some governments have already taken steps to regulate the drug industry so as to attenuate the side-effects of drug promotion and to decrease the use of certain drugs where more effective ones are available.

In conclusion, the uneven distribution of world drug consumption is associated with uneven distribution of drug production, which is concentrated in a few developed countries. The large companies oriented towards research and development play a key role in production and continue to dominate the world market. However, the success of the generics in the United States market is a new development that may bring about changes in the pharmaceutical market in the next ten years, not only in developed but also in developing countries, since it will increase the global availability of low-cost drugs.

As in the past, research has been carried out mainly on the diseases of the developed world. New drugs are still badly needed to combat the health problems of the developing countries. As the cost of research is increasing, there is a trend in the pharmaceutical industry to concentrate on fewer research projects with prospects of greatest profit; as a result, research in specific tropical diseases receives relatively low priority. Some positive changes have been seen in the promotional practices of the industry, although there is still an urgent need to provide complete and unbiased information on drugs to all concerned — governments, prescribers, and consumers.

PART II

The situation
in countries

Introduction

Analysis of the world drug situation shows clearly that the geographical distribution and concentration of drug production and consumption have not changed much in the last decade. The figures are too general, however, to reveal improvements at country level through, for example, a better use of scarce resources or more training of health workers in the rational use of drugs. Many countries have in fact taken steps to impose some order on the prevailing confusion in the use of drugs.

Part II of this report describes the situation in countries on the basis of country reports, discussions with nationals and WHO staff in the countries and regions, national and international publications, etc. The information has been carefully checked, but many data are lacking or are not precise. For future reports, improved methods of collecting quantified information will be used, so that a more accurate description can be given of the situation in countries.

Indicators have been chosen to reflect the progress made by countries towards achieving the objectives of a national drug policy. Like all indicators, those selected for this study measure a complex situation only in part, but they can serve as a basis for comparison of countries at a given moment in time and provide an overall view of the drug situation in countries. Changes in these indicators over time can also indicate progress and the rate of change. The indicators chosen reflect the availability of essential drugs, the extent to which drugs are used rationally, and progress towards improvement. The indicators are not extremely sensitive in all situations; in some countries — mainly the developed ones — it would have been useful to go beyond the indicators to measure with precision such an objective as the rational use of drugs. The indicators must therefore be seen as a starting-point for evaluating progress, and have not been applied to developed countries.

The indicators for the availability of essential drugs of good quality at low cost are:

— the existence and use of an essential drugs list;

— the extent of an operating system for procurement and distribution;

— the extent of quality assurance and regulatory mechanisms;

— the extent of coverage, i.e., the proportion of people in need of essential drugs who actually receive them regularly, including physical, economic, and cultural accessibility. Precise information on this indicator is extremely difficult to obtain, hence broad categories have been used: less than 30%, 30–60%, and 60–90%.

Indicators for the rational use of drugs are also difficult to identify. As it is not possible to quantify rational use *per se*, it has been assumed that certain mechanisms tend to have an influence on the use of drugs. Rational use is then measured by the existence of those mechanisms, i.e.,

— a functioning system that regularly provides objective information on drugs to health workers and patients;

— a system of continuing education for all types of personnel dealing with drugs; and

— a monitoring system, covering adverse drug reactions, and post-marketing surveillance.

The indicators for the development of national pharmaceutical production potential have been taken, slightly revised, from UNIDO. They permit an overview of the type of production in each country and are used to a lesser extent to monitor progress.

A single indicator has been used to provide information on the commitment of the government: is the government interested in the development of a national drug policy, is this policy already at an early stage of development, or is there a strong explicit or implicit national drug policy?

Each indicator is divided into two, three or four levels.[1] Thus a country allocated to level 1 in legislation is a country with a non-functioning drug regulatory administration and outdated legislation, while a country with a coverage at level 3 would be a country where between 60% and 90% of the population have access to essential drugs. Thus the situation in each country can be described (Annex 2) and one can obtain an overview of the general situation in relation to drug coverage, drug policy, legislation, list of essential drugs, etc., prevailing in the 104 developing countries for which information was available. In the following steps, these countries are divided into three groups, according to the availability of essential drugs to their population:

group A: countries where less than 30% of the population has regular access to essential drugs;

group B: countries where 30–60% of the population has regular access to essential drugs;

group C: countries where 60–90% of the population has regular access to essential drugs.

The developed countries are considered separately as group D.

---

[1] See Annex 1 for a definition of each level for each indicator.

This grouping is not meant to suggest that countries develop in a predictable way, since the mechanisms and approaches employed will vary depending on the socioeconomic policy and cultural setting; nevertheless, some issues are common. In each group the situation is described at group level as well as, when necessary, at country level.

This part is divided into five chapters. Chapter 4 provides a general overview of the countries reviewed, based on a broad analysis of the indicators. Chapter 5 focuses on countries where the population has very little access to essential drugs (group A), identifies problems for each indicator, and summarizes action taken by governments to improve the situation. Two countries are described in detail, as they have developed strong policies at national level representing two different strategies aimed at self-sufficiency in the field of drugs.

Along the same lines, Chapter 6 describes the situation in countries where the population has moderate access to essential drugs (group B). Many of these countries have an essential drugs programme, and one is discussed in greater depth. Chapter 7 assesses the situation in the countries in group C, where the population has relatively good access to essential drugs. As the countries are very diverse and have developed different strategies to reach their objectives, three countries are given more thorough study. Chapter 8 sets out the main issues faced by developed countries and the action taken by governments.

The conclusion reviews the main issues, the challenges countries are facing, and some prospects for the future.

Chapter 4

The overall situation

Of the 5 billion people in the world, between 1.3 and 2.5 billion have little or no regular access to essential drugs. These figures are based on the facts that, in 23% of the developing countries reviewed, less than 30% of the population have regular access to essential drugs; in 32% of the countries, between 30% and 60% of the population have access to essential drugs; and in 45% of countries, 60–90% have access (Table 21 and Annex 2). The needs of most of the 1.2 billion people living in developed countries are mostly fulfilled.

Table 21. Distribution of 104 developing countries according to selected indicators (see Annexes 1 and 2)[a]

Level	Policy (%)	Legislation (%)	Essential drugs list (%)	Procurement (%)	Distribution (%)	Coverage (%)	Quality assurance (%)	Information (%)	Manpower development (%)	Monitoring (%)
1	29	25	11	37	36	23	15	55	94	68
2	41	27	45	40	41	32	29	40	4	20
3	25	39	44	20	17	45	43	–	–	7
4	–	5	–	–	–	–	9	–	–	–
Data not available	5	4	–	3	6	–	4	5	2	5

[a] Source: WHO secretariat.

The difference in coverage between countries is largely related to their financial situation, but this does not always provide a sufficient explanation. Policies and their implementation vary from one country to another, giving rise to a wide variety of situations. For example, 25% of countries have a well defined national drug policy, 41% are currently developing a policy aiming at a better availability of essential drugs, and 29% are either considering implementing some kind of essential drugs policy or have no interest in such a policy.

Although many of the 104 countries show an apparent lack of willingness to adopt a strong and effective drug policy, a majority have drug legislation as well as an essential drugs list. Over 65% have legislation that has been classified at level 2 or 3, i.e., they have a drug regulatory administration but it is not fully functioning. Nearly 90% have a revised essential drugs list by generic name at level 2 or 3. However, as will be seen in more detail in the following chapters, many countries do not have the capacity to enforce legislation and/or essential drug lists.

As regards the procurement and distribution of drugs, the situation is more clear-cut; about 80% of the countries have been classified under level 1 or 2, which means that only a minority have a proper system of procurement and distribution. This result is not unexpected in view of the limited infrastructure in many developing countries, their lack of experience in the field of international procurement, and the weakness of their situation on the international scene. This makes it all the more remarkable that, despite the unfavourable environment, 20% of developing countries have a functioning and adequate procurement and distribution system.

Quality control exists in most countries. More than 70% of the 104 coun-tries have some mechanisms for assessing the quality of products or have a quality control laboratory. However, in many of them, this control does not function effectively.

The rational use of drugs remains an area where progress is needed. There is no good system for providing objective information. In most countries, adverse reactions are not monitored and continuing education is not carried out systematically (94% of the countries are at level 1 for this indicator). For many of the Third World countries, the main issue is still how to improve the availability of essential drugs; rational use does not appear to many governments to be a priority.

Chapter 5

Group A: Countries with low coverage

Out of the 104 developing countries reviewed, 24 belong to this first group and are characterized by low coverage, less than 30% of the population having regular access to essential drugs. This means that of the total population of 1.2 billion, over 840 million have no regular access to essential drugs.

The per capita gross domestic product in these countries varies between US$ 130 (Bangladesh) and US$ 810 (Cameroon), most being below 400 dollars; they are thus among the poorest countries in the world. Of their population, over 75% live in rural areas, and agricultural productivity is low. A high percentage of the population is illiterate. The health situation is characterized by severe shortages of such basic requisites as adequate sanitation, safe drinking-water, appropriate nutrition, and adequate health services. Immunization coverage is insufficient, life expectancy at birth is less than 50 years, and infant mortality rates are high. The major causes of morbidity and mortality are preventable communicable diseases and diseases arising out of malnutrition.

The health sector generally consists of a heterogeneous mixture of public and private services, provided by both modern and traditional practition-ers. Although the primary health care strategy has been endorsed by all these countries, modern care is still curative in orientation and is more developed in cities, where most of the facilities and doctors are to be found. In Bangladesh in 1984 there was 1 doctor per 2432 inhabitants in urban areas, as against 1 per 14 382 in rural areas. An infrastructure capable of delivering primary health care services exists in most countries, although at various stages of development, but there is a general lack of the resources needed for effective services, including immunization, vector control, health education, simple curative care and referral, and drug treatment. This is why indigenous systems of medicine are still an important part of the health care system and are used by the majority of the population; in India almost 80% of the population still depend on the Ayurvedic and Unani systems.

The situation in the drug sector is much influenced by the economic situation. Because of the lack of infrastructure, resources, and management capabilities, over 80% of these countries have a poor distribution system, over 65% an inefficient procurement system, and over 35% no mechanism whatsoever for quality control; and none has a drug information service or continuing education (see Table 22 and Annex 2).

The only positive aspect of the situation shown in Table 22 is that most countries have an essential drugs list, either at level 2 (50%) or at level 3 (13%).

The 24 countries are not alike in their attitude to a national drug policy. Ten are at level 1, i.e., either they have no interest in developing a national drug policy or they have an interest but no steps have been taken to improve the situation. Nine have already embarked upon developing a drug policy. Two have a well established national policy. No information is available on three countries.

Table 22.   Distribution of countries in group A (low coverage) according to selected indicators[a, b]

Level	Policy (%)	Legislation (%)	Essential drugs list (%)	Procurement (%)	Distribution (%)	Coverage (%)	Quality assurance (%)	Information (%)	Manpower development (%)	Monitoring (%)
1	42	42	25	67	83	100	38	88	88	75
2	38	29	50	13	4	–	21	–	–	8
3	8	17	13	4	–	–	29	–	–	–
4	–	–	–	–	–	–	–	–	–	–
Data not available	12	12	12	16	13	–	12	12	12	17

[a] Source: WHO secretariat.

[b] For more details see Annexes 1 and 2.

Countries with little or no interest in developing a national drug policy

The characteristics of the countries with little or no interest in developing a national drug policy have been described in numerous reports. Scarcity of financial resources and absence of an adequate infrastructure for the distribution and procurement of drugs create a situation where drug shortages in the public sector are frequent. Public and private systems for distribution of medicines generally exist side by side but the relative size of the two varies considerably. In the public sector, there is a list of a limited number of drugs that are available; this list has recently been updated in Afghanistan, Liberia, Madagascar, Rwanda, and Somalia. In the other countries, the lists have not been revised for a long time and often contain a number of products listed under brand names, and many of doubtful therapeutic value. Needs for drugs are not known and procurement is based on unreliable data on consumption. Even when a tendering system exists, it cannot be used, as funds and foreign exchange are inadequate and provided erratically. Purchases are mainly made directly overseas and from local suppliers at high prices. Stock in hand is sparse, unorganized, and not checked for redundancy, obsolescence, or expiry. Distribution is hampered by lack of vehicles, fuel, and personnel and underdevelopment of the infrastructure. Drugs may stay in the central warehouse or in port for months.

In the private sector a broad range of drugs is generally available. In some rare cases, as in Mauritania before mid-1987, there is no registration of drugs and any product can be imported freely. In most other countries suppliers are required to pay a fee and provide information, but there is neither a functioning drug regulatory agency, nor enough trained personnel, nor explicit scientific criteria for meaningful registration of the drugs. This lack of regulation leads to the marketing and promotion of dangerous and useless products and of drugs that do not meet the health needs of the population (see Chapter 2). Because it is impossible to enforce control over distribution, prescription drugs are frequently sold over the counter and dispensed by untrained retailers. Since the pharmacies procure drugs mainly through wholesalers who have a monopoly of the market, prices are high. In some countries of West Africa, for example, pharmaceutical products are more expensive than in Western Europe and therefore too costly for most of the population; thus, pharmacies are usually situated in the large towns where most of the country's wealth is concentrated. For reasons of economy and geography, therefore, essential drugs are not available to the majority of the population; and even for the few that are available, there is no good system of quality assurance. In the Côte d'Ivoire, Rwanda and Senegal, some control mechanisms are used, such as monitoring of suppliers and occasional testing. Afghanistan puts strong emphasis on reaching self-sufficiency in the local production and quality control of drugs, and there, the quality control laboratory and the Avicenna Pharmaceutical Institute (a semigovernmental production plant for essential drugs) have benefited from WHO support since 1982.

Although shortages are common, overprescribing is frequent and well documented, and is mainly due to lack of continuing education, of objective scientific information on drugs, and of relevant reference material. The only source of information is the pharmaceutical industry.

Interestingly enough, although all these countries import up to 90% of their drugs as finished products, they all, with the exception of Mauritania, have some kind of production facility and are at stage 2 of UNIDO's revised classification, i.e., production of drugs from pharmaceutical chemicals (see Annex 2). A very small part of this production is undertaken by multinational companies for the local private market, the rest being carried out by government-owned companies, such as Istituto Farmaceutico Somalo (IFS) in Somalia, or by a joint venture between the private and the public sector, such as SIPOA in Senegal. Many of these companies encounter various problems, and they are often run with the technical support of a foreign company. Their prices are generally higher than those on the international market and are often beyond the reach of the public sector.

The situation in this small group of countries is partly the result of factors outside the health sector. The countries demonstrate all the classical features of underdevelopment, and the present economic crisis is far from improving the situation. The weakness of political commitment to a primary health care strategy is a limiting factor in solving the main issue, which is how to improve the availability of a limited number of essential drugs at low cost. In many of the countries (Benin, Cameroon, Somalia), local projects funded by external organizations (nongovernmental organizations, bilateral agencies, missions) provide the population with essential drugs, but their coverage is limited and their ability to sustain their actions in the long term precarious as long as procurement of drugs at national level is in disarray. Some of these projects have cost recovery schemes, i.e., drugs are bought cheaply from agencies such as UNICEF, IDA (International Dispensary Association), ECHO (Supply of Equipment to Charity Hospitals Overseas), MEDEOR, etc. and sold to the community. To be viable in the future without foreign aid, the community will have to buy from the national procurement agencies, which at present have prices that are too high for patients in the rural areas.

Some of the countries of this group are interested in improving their drug supply. In Rwanda a national workshop was organized in 1982 with the assistance of WHO and made recommendations on steps to improve the situation. Some of the recommendations have been carried out, for example the formation of a national committee on drugs and one on therapeutics, but the situation governing the supply and use of drugs is still very similar to what it was in 1980 and the concept of a drug policy is not yet well established. Other countries, such as Benin, Madagascar, and Mauritania, with the assistance of international organizations (UNICEF, the World Bank, WHO, the African Development Bank), are assessing their pharmaceutical sector but as yet have taken no decisions on its final form. In all the countries in this group, the private sector (pharmacists and doctors) is very often opposed to an essential drugs policy and, as it is an important and vocal group, the government often has problems in developing a clear-cut policy.

Countries already planning a drug policy

Among the countries with a very low coverage, a second subgroup comprises countries that are already planning a drug policy, although it is at a very early stage.

Most of the characteristics of the first subgroup apply equally to the second. The countries have lists of essential drugs but, with the exception of Angola, Nepal, and Sudan, do not systematically use them for procurement. They procure their drug supplies through tenders, but often have problems because of lack of foreign exchange. Their procurement systems generally need strengthening. In all countries distribution is a major problem; in some (e.g., Angola and Sudan), the problem is aggravated by the presence of guerrillas in certain areas. Bolivia, Nigeria, the Philippines, and Sudan each have a quality control laboratory and a drug regulatory authority, but these authorities have often emphasized the need for further training of staff, including training in management. They have also stressed the importance of improving the enforcement of laws and administrative orders regulating the registration, manufacture, and distribution of drugs.

As drugs are often out of stock in the health facilities, many patients obtain what they need in private pharmacies or through drug sellers who, in general, have no formal training. In Nepal, however, some training courses are organized for drug retailers and a handbook on drugs is available to them.

The number of drugs available in the private sector is considerable (over 10 000 in the Philippines, 15 000 in Nigeria). Irrational prescribing habits further aggravate the problem; prescriptions for up to six drugs are not rare in countries such as Nepal or the Philippines, where doctors are heavily bombarded by promotional materials and free samples. The indiscriminate use of antibiotics is leading to drug resistance; for example the Philippines has the second highest prevalence of gonorrhoea strains resistant to high doses of penicillin. Little information is available to health personnel and the public, other than that supplied by the drug industry. No independent drug bulletins exist, and there is no machinery for the national drug regulatory board to report on adverse drug reactions and other problems.

Under the pressure of the economic crisis, which has further depressed the already meagre budgets of ministries of health, persistent droughts (in Mali and Sudan), the drop in the price of oil (Angola and Nigeria) and changes in the political situation (Bolivia, Guinea and the Philippines), the countries in the group are beginning to develop more rational drug policies.

Mali and Nepal, with the support of various international organizations, have for a few years been reorganizing their pharmaceutical sector

Progress is slow, but the governments have reiterated their support for a national essential drugs policy, lists of essential drugs have been revised and partly used for procurement, and some training has taken place; in Mali the use of tenders has enabled savings of 40% to be made on the prices paid normally. Many problems remain unsolved: improvement of procurement and distribution, strengthening of the drug authority (a quality control laboratory is being installed in Mali with the assistance of the European Economic Community), further training of health workers (the essential drugs concept is still encountering a lot of resistance), and the creation of financial mechanisms to allow the programmes to become self-sustaining.

Since 1986 Angola, Burma, Guinea, Nigeria, and Sudan have embarked on large essential drugs programmes with the objective of ensuring that essential drugs are available at all levels in the health care system. In most cases a step-by-step approach is being adopted with pilot projects in, for example, the Nile Province in Sudan, Imo, Ogun, Oyo and Sokoto States in Nigeria, at township level in Burma, and at operational health centres in Guinea. The programmes entail selection of essential drugs, quantification of needs, improvement of procurement methods, storage, distribution, training of health workers, and establishment of cost-recovery schemes and revolving drug funds. For the next few years these programmes will be funded externally, by direct grants or loans. In the future much will depend on the functioning of the cost-recovery schemes and on the ability of the governments to provide sufficient foreign exchange on a regular basis. In the meantime, the necessary support mechanisms for an essential drugs programme have to be developed, mainly in relation to regulation of pharmaceutical drug registration, drug procurement, provision of information, and quality assurance.

In the Philippines, the President has announced a new national drug policy, which will focus on four main areas: expansion and strengthening of the role of the regulatory authority; systematization of government procurement activities, employing such measures as bulk purchasing, active participation in production, and improving the national distribution network for rural health units and hospitals; provision of adequate information on drugs for both doctors and patients; and coordination of investment and trade policies to achieve self-sufficiency in pharmaceuticals. Among the measures planned are the elaboration of a national formulary to control the proliferation of products, the introduction of generic labelling, the removal of banned, harmful and ineffective drugs from the market, and the enforcement of policies on pharmaceutical advertising and promotion.

All the countries of this subgroup are at stage 2 of the revised UNIDO classification, although the extent of local production differs greatly from one to the other. In both Nigeria and the Philippines there are over 100 drug manufacturers, while in the other countries there are fewer than

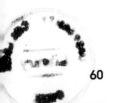

five. In all of them the main issue is how to stimulate the growth of cost-effective local production geared to the health needs of the population so that essential drugs are made available at a reasonable cost.

The next five years will be of crucial importance for these countries as regards the availability of drugs for their population. The way to success is full of pitfalls and the opposition is substantial, but success can still be achieved as long as the level of political commitment remains high.

Countries with a well defined drug policy

Bangladesh and India share a number of features with the other countries in this group, mainly in the field of distribution, quality control, and use, but they differ from the others in having well defined national drug policies. These will be described in more detail as they represent two different strategies aimed at self-sufficiency in the field of drugs.

India

India is characterized by a strong pharmaceutical industry capable of manufacturing nearly all the drugs needed in the country. According to UNIDO, India is in category 4, i.e., technologically developed enough to be totally self-reliant, with research capability for the discovery of new chemical entities.

The responsibility for the pharmaceutical sector is shared between two ministries: the Ministry of Industry, Department of Chemicals and Petro-chemicals which deals with the new drug policy, prices and profits, technology, etc., and the Ministry of Health and Family Welfare, which deals with registration and quality control.

With the advent of independence, the Government planned an orderly integrated growth of the pharmaceutical industry in India. The 1956 industrial policy resolution set the tempo for industrialization, with emphasis on self-reliance. On the basis of some of the recommendations made by the Hathi Committee in 1975, a national drug policy was proclaimed in 1978 with the following objectives: to develop self-reliance in drug technology; to accord a leadership role to the public sector; to achieve self-sufficiency in the production of 117 essential drugs and thus reduce the level of imports; to encourage the growth of the domestic sector; to ensure that drugs are available in abundance and at a reasonable price to meet the health needs of the people; to maintain high standards of production; and to promote research and development. Among other measures it was decided that importation of the necessary raw materials would be carried out on behalf of the manufacturers by the State Trading Corporation (STC), a process known as "drug canalization". The imported raw materials were pooled with raw materials produced domestically by the government-owned Indian Drugs and Pharmaceuticals Limited, and the pooled stock was then distributed to manufacturers in both the public and the private sector. The objectives of canalization were to prevent transfer-pricing and to ensure a reliable supply of raw materials to indigenous manufacturers at a fair price.

Since the report of the Hathi Committee in 1975 and the promulgation of the drug policy in 1978, there have been significant changes in the pharmaceutical industry. The production of finished products reached a value of 20 billion rupees (Rs) in 1985–86, that of bulk drugs 4 billion rupees. A cumulative growth of 19.6% from 1971–72 to 1978–79 in formulation and 22% in bulk drugs took place. Imports of finished formulations (tablets, injections, etc., ready packed for retail sale) have been virtually eliminated. Drug exports have increased. All this has produced net savings in foreign exchange.

However, the 1978 policy has not achieved all the intended results. Between 1952 and 1983 the number of production units grew 3-fold, investment 24-fold, and bulk drug production 18-fold. Yet the production of essential drugs in 1980 accounted for only Rs 3.5 billion of an overall total production worth Rs 12.6 billion. Imports of bulk drugs, mostly essential, reached a record Rs 1.78 billion in 1984–85, about half of the indigenous production. In the five years between 1978–79 and 1983–84 the industry's sales of essential drugs with the lowest price mark-up actually dipped from Rs 554.7 million to Rs 493.5 million, while sales of other drugs for which the Government permits higher mark-ups grew by over 25% – from Rs 1544.4 million to Rs 1983.8 million. In the absence of any specific requirement that essential drugs should be produced, companies concentrated on the more profitable non-priority end of the market. As a result, essential drugs are in short supply in many parts of the country; in 1980 they constituted 16.8% of the total of drugs consumed. Tonics, vitamins, restoratives, and enzyme preparations constitute 25% of the drugs in the market.

To step up production in general and boost stagnating drug exports, the Government adjusted its policy in 1986. Among the changes were: the introduction of a new comprehensive pricing system; changes in licensing policy; decanalization of imported raw materials and intermediates; and the maximum priority to making essential drugs available. Requirements for the registration of new drugs will be revised and the marketing of new drugs will not be allowed unless they can be demonstrated to possess distinct advantages over existing products. However, because of the complexity of implementing national drug policies, although India has strict and comprehensive legislation on the import, manufacture and sale of drugs, much remains to be done to implement the reforms.

To improve the availability of essential drugs, measures to regulate prices have previously been taken by the Government, culminating in the Drug Price Control Order (DPCO) of 1970. However, pharmaceutical firms took advantage of some aspects of the Order and increased the prices of unregulated drugs to compensate for the control. To remedy the situation, a new order was issued in 1979, dividing formulations or finished products of 37 bulk drugs into three categories according to their "essentiality", with a different price mark-up for each category. Unfortunately the policy led to the adoption of price control measures that proved difficult to implement in practice.

With the 1986 drug policy, all bulk drugs and their formulations have been freed from price control except for a priority list of 166 bulk drugs, which fall into two price-controlled categories. The mark-up on finished drugs in controlled categories I and II increased respectively from 40% and 55% to 75% and 100% of manufacturing costs. Small units with turnovers of under Rs 5 million will continue to be exempt from price control. Finished drugs in category II, produced by companies with investments totalling less than Rs 3.5 million, are also exempt from price control. All single-ingredient formulations sold under generic names have also been freed from price control. Production of these drugs and their formulations should, subject to government monitoring, account for 20% of the total output in value of every manufacturer in India. The new Drug Price Control Order was issued in August 1987. As for the critical question of ensuring that prices are under control, a monitoring system, the National Drug and Pharmaceutical Authority (NDPA), will be set up, but is not likely to be functional for at least a year and at best will be only an advisory body. This new pricing policy could improve the availability of essential drugs, though at a higher cost – anything from 13% to 43% above current prices. Some sources predict a possible increase in cost of 50–300%. On the other hand, the argument has been put forward that a differential mark-up for finished products combined with price controls for a selected few (leaving the rest to be sold in the open market without strict price control) will encourage the industry to produce more non-essential drugs and also increase their prices. Already, prior to the new Drug Price Control Order, the prices of all drugs showed a 30% mark-up and drug company shares were selling at a premium. This is despite the fact that the drug controllers were instructed to ensure that there was no price increase before the issuance of the Order.

Although drug prices have not risen as much as the prices of other commodities in India, the increase has been substantial. The drug price index rose from 135.2 in 1979–80 to 167 in 1982–84. Thus, despite price control and the phenomenal growth of the drug industry during the last three decades, the availability of modern drugs is still very low. For example, in 1984 only 5–6% of the population were able to afford or procure the modern drugs they needed; another 25% had limited access to essential drugs. A majority of the people living in rural areas and urban slums, the main victims of endemic and epidemic diseases, had no or very little access to modern drugs. With the predicted increase in the cost of drugs, the problems are likely to be accentuated.

As well as the lack of the most basic drugs for entire groups of the population, there is a proliferation on the market of formulations without adequate therapeutic rationale. Concern has been expressed in several Indian newspapers regarding harmful and/or ineffective formulations, in particular combination drugs such as antibiotics plus vitamins, penicillin plus streptomycin, chloramphenicol plus streptomycin, and various cough syrups containing ingredients with opposing effects. More than 20 000 combination drugs are on the market. The indiscriminate use of antibiotics has led to the development of bacterial drug resistance; thus multiresistant *Salmonella typhimurium* infection has spread all over India, causing serious outbreaks in hospitals and nurseries.

However, towards the end of 1987, the Drugs Technical Advisory Board, a statutory body established under the Drugs and Cosmetics Act, recommended that the Central Government ban a large number of these irrational formulations. It is understood that the Government has now effectively done so, an action that is likely to weed out a large number of harmful and hazardous combinations.

Consumer organizations, under the auspices of the All India Drug Action Network, are growing in strength and are distributing drug information packets to doctors. In most instances, however, medical information from representatives of pharmaceutical companies is the only source of information to prescribers in remote areas.

From this brief description of what has happened in India in the last twenty years it is evident that it is not always possible to reconcile economic and health goals. India provides a paradoxical example of overproduction of drugs existing simultaneously with shortage of essential drugs for major diseases. Although attempts have been made by the Hathi Committee to elaborate a policy geared to meeting the health needs of the people, this policy has not been followed completely and economic priorities have often taken precedence over health priorities. The new policy is an attempt to redress the situation and ensure availability of essential medicines for everyone. It is, however, too early as yet to assess its impact.

Bangladesh

In Bangladesh in 1982 a new drug policy and supplementary drug legislation (the Drug Control Ordinance, 1982) were promulgated, which *inter alia* provide administrative and legislative support for ensuring the quality and availability of essential drugs, reducing the price of drugs and raw materials, eliminating useless, non-essential and harmful drugs from the market, promoting local production, and developing a drug monitoring and information system.

A committee appointed by the Ministry of Health developed a set of guidelines to evaluate all registered/licensed pharmaceutical products manufactured in or imported into Bangladesh, Nearly all combination products were to be withdrawn, unless there was absolutely no alternative single drug available for treatment. The sale of tonics and of some duplicate drugs was prohibited. Doubtful and harmful drugs were banned. Drugs and raw materials produced in Bangladesh were not allowed to be imported. Multinational companies were not allowed to produce antacids and vitamins. Under these guidelines, out of a total of about 4000 brands of registered allopathic drugs, the registration or licence of 1701 brands of locally manufactured or imported drugs was cancelled. This procedure took longer than planned because of the pressures put on the Government by a number of interested parties. A list of 150 essential drugs by generic name was drawn up for the national health system. A supplementary list of 100 was established for restricted use by specialists.

As a result of the new policy, in 1984 over 80% of the country's requirements for drugs were produced locally. Almost all raw materials were imported. About 2300 locally manufactured products and 1600 foreign products were registered and authorized for marketing in Bangladesh. Only drugs that have been approved and registered by the Bangladesh Drug Administration can be imported into the country.

One of the objectives of the drug policy was to save foreign exchange previously spent on the import of irrelevant, dangerous, or overpriced products. This was achieved by removing certain products from the market, purchasing products on the world market at competitive prices, and carrying out careful investigation of requests for registration of imported drugs by pharmaceutical companies. The total cost of imports of raw materials in local currency approximately doubled between 1981 and 1985, from 451 to 982 million taka (approximately US$ 22.5 million to US$ 32.7 million) (Table 23), but the average price paid in 1986 for a number of raw materials was lower than in 1981; for instance, the price of ampicillin was US$ 75 per kg in 1985 against US$ 120 in 1981, doxycycline cost US$ 175 instead of US$ 1500, rifampicin US$ 230 against US$ 473, and mebendazole US$ 52 against US$ 287. Thus, far more drugs were being produced per dollar spent on imports. Imports of finished products

65

Table 23.   Value of imports of drugs to Bangladesh, 1981–85[a, b]

	Value (millions of taka)				
	1981	1982	1983	1984	1985
Pharmaceutical raw materials	451	487	676	952	982
Packing materials	127	132	165	230	245
Finished drugs	284	270	232	300	337
Total	862	889	1073	1482	1564
	(43.1)[c]	(40.4)[c]	(42.9)[c]	(52.9)[c]	(52.1)[c]

[a] Source: ISLAM, N. & CHOUDHURY, S.A.R., ed. *Proceedings of the Conference on Essential Drugs in Primary Health Care, Dhaka, February 4-9, 1986.*

[b] Does not include the D & D kits received from UNICEF.

[c] Figure in parentheses gives the equivalent value in millions of US$.

(284 million taka in 1981, 337 million in 1985) have not risen as fast as raw materials, and more products are now manufactured locally.

In 1982 the market was dominated by eight multinational companies producing about 75% of the market share, followed by 25 medium-sized companies producing 15%, while other companies accounted for the remaining 10%. The Government today has a larger share in the pharmaceutical industry, as full or part owner. The share of production by Bangladeshi corporations rose from 35.3% of total local production in 1981 to 54.2% in 1985 (Table 24). Production of the first 45 essential drugs doubled between 1981 and 1983 and represented 56% of total local production in 1983 as against 30% in 1981. The share of this production by national companies was 80% (Tables 25 and 26).

Table 24.   Share of Bangladeshi companies in local drug production, 1981–85[a]

	Value (millions of taka)				
	1981	1982	1983	1984	1985
Total local production	1730	2160	2260	2830	3200
Production of Bangladeshi companies (% of total)	613 (35.3%)	842 (39.0%)	1160 (51.3%)	1470 (52.0%)	1680 (54.2%)

[a] Source: HYE, H. *The Bangladesh experience.* Presented at *Medicines and society*, a multidisciplinary course on rational use of drugs, Stockholm, 1987. For more details, write to Action Programme on Essential Drugs, World Health Organization, 1211 Geneva 27, Switzerland.

Table 25. Production of essential drugs in Bangladesh by multi-national and national companies[a]

	Multinational companies		National companies	
	Value (millions of taka)	%	Value (millions of taka)	%
Before 1981				
First 12 essential drugs	116	34	228	66
Next 33 essential drugs	121	67	59	33
Total	237	45	287	55
January–October 1983				
First 12 essential drugs	94	20	388	80
Second 33 essential drugs	145	25	426	75
Total	239	21	814	79

[a] Source: Figures supplied by Minister of Health of Bangladesh at a press conference, 28 December 1983.

Table 26. Production of essential drugs in Bangladesh[a]

	Before 1981		January–October 1983	
	Value (millions of taka)	%	Value (millions of taka)	%
Total production (all drugs)	1734	100	1883	100
First 12 essential drugs	344	20	482	26
Next 33 essential drugs	180	10	571	30
Share of first 45 essential drugs	524	30	1053	56

[a] Source: Figures supplied by the Minister of Health of Bangladesh at a press conference, 28 December 1983.

The monopoly existing in certain therapeutic classes was to a certain extent broken by the new drug policy. When many of the most profitable drugs were banned, the multinational companies were forced to compete in terms of both prices and products. The restriction imposed on the manufacture of vitamins and antacids by the multinational companies provided an opportunity for local companies.

Following initial reservations, the national pharmaceutical companies now have a more positive attitude towards the new drug policy, as reflected in an article by the Bangladesh Association of Pharmaceutical Industry in the newspaper *New nation*, detailing the benefits the industry has reaped from the policy. A letter from the Association in 1986 approved ratification of the Drug Control Ordinance.

Nor have the multinational companies suffered drastically from the new policy. Their output has not declined, and some firms have actually benefited. In all, 170 drugs produced by the multinationals were banned by the Ordinance, but several new drugs produced by them have been approved and others reformulated; more than 136 of these new products are now on the market. The attraction of the pharmaceutical market in Bangladesh has not declined: local companies have expanded, while at the same time the entire pharmaceutical market has grown, thus leaving ample room for the multinational companies too. Since the new drug policy was introduced one more multinational company has entered the market, and there have been no reports of companies intending to leave.

Although there has been remarkable progress in the production of essential drugs, it is still insufficient; 70–80% of the population are without access to even basic essential drugs and, while antibiotics may be available, other fundamental drugs are not. About 10% of drugs are distributed free of charge in the public sector. Only small amounts of drugs reach the health system below the *thana* health complexes, the supplies are irregular, and even the *thana* health complexes are frequently short of essential drugs. An essential drugs programme has been established in one province, with DANIDA support, and will be extended to larger areas.

The remaining 90% of drugs are sold by 14 000 retailers. The Drug Ordinance states that all retail sales of drugs must be under the supervision of a pharmacist, but owing to the lack of pharmacists and the understaffing of the drug administration this has proved difficult in practice.

The maximum retail price of drugs is decided by the Government under the Essential Commodities Act, but enforcement of the Act is weak. However, despite the pressure of inflation, the market price of some essential drugs has been reduced since the new policy came into force because of increased competition, control of prices of raw materials, and the prohibition of the manufacture of a drug by a company under another company's brand name. Even so, prices are still too high for the majority of the population, whose annual income is less than US$ 100 per capita. The average spending on pharmaceuticals was US$ 1.25 per capita in 1985, one of the lowest in the world. Only the wealthier 20% of the population have easy access to drugs and health care. Polypharmacy is widespread, the average number of drugs on each prescription being four. Doctors' knowledge of drugs still often depends on information provided by companies and their representatives; loyalty to brand-name products is strong and prevents essential drugs, especially generic ones, from being used more widely.

Two other areas are of concern in Bangladesh: quality control and traditional medicines. Quality control capacity is very limited and the drug administration is too understaffed to exercice adequate control. Drug sample tests in 1983 and 1985 showed some improvement in the quality of products, 18.6% of samples being unacceptable in 1983 as against 10.7% in 1985. Nevertheless, the number of substandard products is high. DANIDA, with WHO assistance, is supporting the Ministry of Health in this field.

Before the new drug policy traditional medicines were uncontrolled. Under the Ordinance, a large number of these medicines were banned, but enforcement of the policy on Ayurvedic and Unani drugs was postponed several times, the Ministry of Health having only slight control over the producing companies. Because of this lack of control the manufacture of traditional medicines has become an attractive investment prospect: the number of units manufacturing Unani and Ayurvedic drugs increased from 151 in 1978 and 1981 to 336 in 1986. This has led to the production of drugs of doubtful efficacy, several of which are claimed to have the same curative potential as banned drugs. Evidence shows that some of these drugs have been packaged and marketed in such a way as to appear to be substitutes for the banned drugs.

In conclusion, the Bangladesh drug policy has in a few years permitted several steps forward to be taken in lowering prices, controlling transfer pricing, increasing essential drug production, stimulating local companies, and removing dangerous drugs from the market. However, the Government still faces a number of obstacles to the success of the policy. While it is making efforts to ensure that essential drugs are made available to the majority of the population, the Government realizes that it needs to strengthen the health sector and, in particular, the drug administration, including quality control. There is also an awareness of the need to improve control of the production of traditional medicines. Attempts to overcome the various obstacles are hampered by the scanty resources available to the Government.

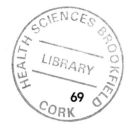

Chapter 6

Group B: Countries with medium coverage

This second group comprises 33 developing countries in which between 30% and 60% of the population has regular access to essential drugs. Thus between 280 million and 490 million of the total population of 700 million have no regular access to essential drugs.

The level of economic development in these countries is slightly higher than in the countries in group A; the per capita GDP varies from US$ 110 to US$ 1370, with an average of about US$ 600. Economically they are more heterogeneous; a larger number have some industrial capacity, but many depend mainly on the export of basic products, which makes them highly vulnerable to price fluctuations on the world market. They mainly import manufactured goods.

The health situation is characterized by slightly better access to adequate sanitation, safe drinking-water, etc. Infant mortality rates are still often above 100 per thousand live births; life expectancy at birth is below 60 years in 26 countries. Communicable diseases remain the major causes of mortality and morbidity, but chronic diseases are emerging.

The health sector has the same characteristics as in group A; it is a mixture of public and private, with a primary health care strategy, but with an imbalance between rural and urban areas, a lack of resources, and the presence of important indigenous systems of medicine. In most of the countries health services are free, but some governments are turning to the community for financial participation. In the Latin American countries, social security systems exist that cover public sector workers and private employees (10–20% of the population), but the self-employed and the rural and economically marginal groups are still categories of the population who are often not covered by these systems.

In the field of drugs, although economic development in some countries may explain the differences in coverage, this is not so for the majority. The main difference from group A is in the level of political commitment. Of the 33 countries, 25 have a national drug policy aimed at improving the availability of essential drugs, 19 are in the early stages of implementing the policy, and six already have a well established policy (Table 27 and Annex 2).

Table 27. Distribution of countries in group B (medium coverage) according to selected indicators [a, b]

Level	Policy (%)	Legislation (%)	Essential drugs list (%)	Procurement (%)	Distribution (%)	Coverage (%)	Quality assurance (%)	Information (%)	Manpower development (%)	Monitoring (%)
1	24	40	6	30	39	–	21	73	97	91
2	58	33	52	58	55	100	36	27	3	3
3	18	27	42	12	3	–	40	–	–	6
4	–	–	–	–	–	–	3	–	–	–
Data not available	–	–	–	–	3	–	–	–	–	–

[a] Source: WHO secretariat.

[b] For more details see Annexes 1 and 2.

However, this political commitment has not always found a concrete expression in legislation. There are still 24 countries, some of which are well advanced in implementing an essential drugs policy, that have outdated legislation and a drug regulatory administration that is not functioning or is taking only the most basic steps. Democratic Yemen till recently had no system of drug registration, but this will be established in 1988 and computerized. Burundi, Uganda and Zaire have just reviewed their legislation. In 1980, Indonesia elaborated criteria for drug evaluation covering safety and efficacy, actual needs, rational dosage forms, strength, and labelling. All drugs registered before 1980 are being re-evaluated in groups, and regulatory action has been taken to ban or limit the use of, for example, some fixed combinations of antibiotics or to correct the labelling. But in all the countries, even in those that have had a drug regulatory administration for many years and a comprehensive drug legislation (e.g., Colombia, Pakistan, Peru, Thailand), enforcement of the laws and regulations is weak owing to the lack of trained personnel, resources, and coordination. In the Latin American countries the impact of the economic crisis on salaries in the public sector has deprived regulatory administrations of valuable staff.

Most of the countries in this group, with the exception of Viet Nam, have large private markets. The situation is characterized by high prices for drugs, proliferation of branded products (6000 in Colombia, 7000 in Pakistan, 12 000 in Indonesia, 20 000 in Thailand), overabundance of non-essential drugs such as vitamins, tonics, and cough syrups, the presence of unsafe drugs, inconsistency of information, absence of objective information for the prescriber and the patient, overconsumption in some sectors of the population, and widespread irrational drug use.

In the field of quality assurance the same cheerless picture can be drawn. Nearly half of the countries have a quality control laboratory, but none functions optimally. Some countries with local production and a large pharmaceutical private market, such as Colombia, rely on university laboratories. To try to improve the situation in Latin America, WHO has organized a network of the existing quality control laboratories, to facilitate the exchange of information, promote collaboration between countries, permit the organization of joint training sessions, etc. In the African Region, three WHO regional quality control laboratories will be set up to serve mainly as reference laboratories. Indonesia is already well advanced in this field with a stratified network of quality control laboratories, including one at national level and 27 at provincial level; a referral scheme has been developed between the different classes of laboratory. About 75 000 samples of drugs are taken annually from the market and analysed. Drug manufacturers are regularly supervised by drug inspectors to ensure that they observe good manufacturing practices.

While legislation and quality assurance are generally at a low level in this group, all the countries except two have an essential drugs list, by generic names, which is new or has recently been revised. In most cases only products on this list can be prescribed in the public sector. The list is divided into sublists for each level of use. National lists comprise from 150 dosage forms (Democratic Yemen) to 300 (Honduras, Indonesia) and to 400–500 (Morocco, Pakistan, Thailand, Yemen). In 40% of the countries, drug requirements, mainly for the primary and secondary levels of care, are calculated according to morbidity data and standard treatments, rather than on unreliable data on previous consumption.

The higher level of political commitment compared with group A is well shown by the procurement and distribution systems. The majority of group B countries are at level 2, i.e., the procurement systems and distribution networks operate fairly well, and prices are not too high. There are exceptions to this, some countries having good procurement and low commitment or poor procurement and high commitment. These will be described separately later.

Countries with an essential drugs programme

In the last few years, a large number of countries in group B, with WHO assistance, have embarked on a national essential drugs programme (Bhutan, Burkina Faso, Democratic Yemen, Ethiopia, Ghana, Guinea-Bissau, Malawi, Mozambique, Sierra Leone, Uganda, Viet Nam, Zambia, Zimbabwe). In most of the programmes the emphasis is on quantification of drug needs, improvement of storage and distribution through, among other things, a standardized drug supply system (drug ration kits), and national, regional, and district training programmes in the rational management and use of drugs. These essential drugs programmes are generally geared to dispensaries and health centres, but in most countries, planned activities include strengthening of the national essential drugs policy by, for example, establishing a small quality control laboratory, disseminating a guide to treatment, improving the drug registration system, and revising the health training curricula to introduce the concept of essential drugs. One area of concern in most of the programmes is the rational use of drugs. Now that the availability of drugs has been secured, more remains to be done in training health workers.

Many of these programmes are still assisted by bilateral agencies in the form of technical support and supply of drugs. The challenge in the next few years is to develop self-sustaining programmes. To achieve that end, some countries are testing cost-recovery schemes, which can only partly solve the problem as they do not deal with the issue of scarcity of foreign exchange. All are trying to rationalize their entire drug supply system, and ministries of health are seeking to improve their negotiating power vis-à-vis the central banks. This is not easy, as these countries are among the poorest in the world. Zimbabwe will be described in more detail as it is fairly representative of this group of countries.

Zimbabwe

In Zimbabwe at independence the Government committed itself to the attainment of health for all by the year 2000. The primary health care strategy was chosen as the best way of achieving that goal, with special emphasis on immunization, nutrition, education, mother and child care, and child-spacing. A major decision was to keep the budget of the large central hospital static and concentrate on expanding rural health facilities. The 400 existing clinics are currently being raised to rural health centre level, to make appropriate health care more accessible to the rural population. There are plans for the construction of an additional 316 rural health centres, of which half had already been commissioned in 1985. Thousands of village health workers have been trained in basic preventive and curative care and in the provision of health education. Mobile maternal and child health and family planning services have been introduced in rural areas.

Traditional medicine is still a very important alternative to the modern health care system; it is estimated that Zimbabwe has some 20 000 traditional healers. Self-medication is also a common practice; according to one study a significant number of people prefer retail drug outlets to government facilities.

One of the reasons for the success of traditional healers and self-medication is the lack of essential drugs in health facilities. A baseline survey on the availability of essential drugs at different levels was carried out in February 1987 by the Zimbabwean Essential Drugs Action Programme (ZEDAP). It found that, although access to health care facilities was adequate in almost all cases, there was an absolute shortage of essential drugs, more than 50% of the essential drugs being out of stock in the rural health care centres. The situation is not much better in provincial hospitals, where on average 47% of the items requested cannot be supplied. In district hospitals 59% of the items cannot be supplied. The Ministry of Health has a budget of approximately 12 million Zimbabwe dollars (Z$) for the purchase of medical supplies. These are procured through an open tender system, but foreign exchange is scarce, the Ministry of Health in 1986 receiving only Z$ 3 million of foreign exchange out of the Z$ 9.7 million requested. Thus the funds and stocks available in government medical stores are insufficient to cover the orders from the health care facilities. Furthermore, when a supplier has won a tender, it often takes so long to obtain the foreign exchange needed that prices go up in the meantime.

Even when the medical stores have the requested items in stock, the average delivery time is ten weeks. This average covers wide variations according to whether there is a provincial store in the region or not. If there is, it takes 1–4 weeks from the date of requisition to the date of delivery. If there is no medical store, the delay could be much longer. e.g., up to 20 weeks in Manicaland and 16 weeks on average in Mashonaland.

The result of all this is shortage of supplies in the government medical stores, forcing health care facilities to cover their drug needs by buying in the private sector and leaving the bill to be paid by the Ministry of Health. The Government may pay 5–10 times more for drugs in the private market than if they were supplied through the government stores system. The ensuing shortage of funds again leads to further shortage of drugs in the government medical stores. The private sector then takes advantage of this situation to ask for more foreign exchange allocations.

Independently of what it sells to the public sector, the private sector supplies drugs to 20% of the population and in value, represents 60% of drug consumption. An important part of total consumption (40%) is met by local production. There is no production of raw materials, but a well functioning formulating and packing industry.

Eleven companies are engaged in the manufacture of pharmaceuticals; three of these — CAPS, Datlabs, and Gulf Marketing — account for 67% of total production. CAPS, which is 42.6% owned by the Government, manufactures a number of essential drugs and 50% of its turnover goes to the public sector, 30% to the local market, and 20% to the export market.

Of the 37 importers/distributors active in Zimbabwe, 20 are controlled by a CAPS-owned company called GEDDES, which handles about 95% of the pharmaceutical preparations in the country. Many of the big multinational companies are represented by marketing agents in Zimbabwe.

Although drug registration is based on therapeutic and economic criteria, difficulties have been encountered in enforcing the criteria, resulting in a variety of expensive branded products on the market. The need to set up a quality control system has been recognized.

To improve the situation, the Government issued a proposed essential drugs list in 1981. After revision by appropriate bodies and institutions it was published in 1985 as the Essential Drugs List for Zimbabwe (EDLIZ). Zimbabwe has about 2000 drugs registered, but EDLIZ contains only 375. The list applies only to the public sector. It is now mandatory for all government and government-aided institutions to prescribe by generic name only and in accordance with the recommendations in EDLIZ. EDLIZ contains not only a list of essential drugs for all levels of health care (except the specialist level), but also recommendations for the treatment of common medical conditions in Zimbabwe. Drugs not listed in EDLIZ can be prescribed only in special cases, with the permission of the Secretary for Health.

EDLIZ was a valiant attempt to promote the rational use of drugs in Zimbabwe. However, although all facilities visited during the Zimbabwe Essential Drugs Action Programme (ZEDAP) baseline survey were found to have a copy of EDLIZ, it was not being followed to the extent intended. The medical stores receive many requisitions for drugs outside EDLIZ. It is significant that in the ZEDAP survey the personnel's use of EDLIZ was found to be poor and none of the clinical staff had any knowledge about the prices of drugs. From the point of view of prescribing, there seems to be a need for further training in economical prescribing and dispensing, stock control, ordering, and storage.

A training programme for promotion of the rational use of drugs has been drawn up. It includes both special courses on drug management and use and incorporation of these concepts into existing training courses and syllabuses. The training programme, which is planned to be carried out in 1988–89, covers all health care levels. It ranges from community orienta- tion meetings and courses for village health workers to courses for senior staff at the provincial level. Furthermore, ZEDAP will prepare a training manual covering a variety of clinical conditions and drug management and administration.

ZEDAP was launched in April 1987 and a national workshop was held for all those involved. The purpose of the workshop was to formulate a policy on drugs. The policy formulated addresses all the problems identified. Among other things it aims to ensure that only EDLIZ drugs are imported by the public sector. Under this policy all purchases for this sector will be made by the government medical stores. For the importation, manufacture, registration, prescription, and dispensing of drugs, generic names only will be used. To encourage the import of EDLIZ drugs by the private sector, the permitted price mark-up on non-EDLIZ items will be lower than that on EDLIZ items. An ethical code of conduct for drug representatives is to be drawn up in consultation with the organizations involved.

The drug policy also seeks to strengthen the Ministry of Health, especially as regards an increased and regular allocation of foreign exchange for drug purchases. The ZEDAP estimation of drug requirements will be used to calculate allocations of foreign exchange for drug purchases. The Ministry of Health is also to have an influence on health-related purchases by other ministries. Government medical stores are to be allowed a realistic mark-up on their drugs so that overhead costs can be covered. A national stock control and ordering/delivery system will be introduced. For the better management of drugs the pharmaceutical service department will be strengthened by the appointment of several new directors and pharmaceu- tical posts will be established at provincial and district level.

A major component of the new drug policy is support for the local pharmaceutical industry. Incentives will be given to increase the local production of essential drugs so that the country can save foreign exchange and become self-sufficient. The duty and surtax on imported raw materials will be waived or refunded to producers on proof of use for the local production of essential drugs. The extent to which duties and surtax can be imposed on imported non-EDLIZ products will be studied. The production of simple preparations in the public sector will also be encouraged.

In conclusion, Zimbabwe has attempted to shift the emphasis from an élite-centred, curative, sophisticated, urban-based health care system to a majority-oriented, preventive, rural-based primary health care system. Rural health care facilities are now more accessible to the majority of the population, both geographically and economically. Not all the problems have been solved, but the commitment is strong, especially concerning the availability of pharmaceuticals. It may be noted that, although Zimbabwe produced the first draft of an essential drugs list six years ago, the mere existence of the list was not enough to ensure the constant availability of essential drugs to people in the rural areas. If such a list is not incorporated in a national drug policy addressing such crucial issues as procurement, the private sector, drug distribution, and the training of manpower, and if the Ministry of Health is not strong, the desired effect cannot be achieved. This demonstrates that a comprehensive approach is necessary to ensure the availability and rational use of drugs.

Countries with elements of a national drug policy

Other countries in group B have developed elements of a national drug policy. In Latin America, the countries are generally richer (per capita gross domestic product between US$ 700 and US$ 1400), and more money is available for drugs in the public and private sectors. In Central America, Colombia, and Ecuador, per capita expenditure on drugs is between US$ 10 and US$ 15. In this group of countries social security systems cover around 15% of the population, and the ministry of health the remainder; however, often coverage is moderate, procurement very inefficient, lists exist but are different for each institution and contain a large number of products, there is no central purchasing, prices are high, and distribution in the rural areas is deficient. The economic crisis, which has reduced resources, has constrained these countries to adopt an essential drugs programme in an attempt to maintain services with less money; indeed, often it has been necessary to provide more services, as people are poorer and not able to buy the drugs they need in private pharmacies.

Between 1985 and 1987, essential drugs were designated one of the seven priority areas of a comprehensive plan for joint health services action agreed upon by the countries of Central America. Colombia created a national essential drugs fund for the poorest of the population and drew up an essential drugs policy in order to ensure that the money was spent in an efficient way. Ecuador developed a national programme aimed at ensuring a supply of essential drugs free to children below five years of age. Peru launched an initiative aimed at supplying the most remote areas with kits containing 16 drugs.

The objective of the Central American initiative is to increase the availability of quality essential drugs at an accessible price through the improvement of national supply systems and national quality control systems, the framing of coherent national pharmaceutical policies including support for the local production of essential drugs, and the establishment of joint purchasing, using a revolving fund called "Formed". Formed is administered by the Pan American Health Organization/WHO Regional Office for the Americas to facilitate the purchase of drugs in the international market, since prices in Central America are 2–4 times higher than international prices. A list of 18 priority drugs for primary health care was drawn up. In 1985, using this mechanism, the countries saved US$ 1 352 000, paying US$ 2.4 million for drugs that would have cost US$ 3.7 million at regional prices. In addition, an information system on drug prices in the public sector has been set up to create better negotiating positions and disseminate information on alternative suppliers.

In Colombia, the Government has established a fund to ensure the availability of 35 basic drugs as part of its programme for the eradication of absolute poverty. The money will come from taxes. The fund is part of a broader national essential drugs policy, which includes improvement of supply and quality control, development of a national formulary, price control, and promotion of local production.

In Ecuador money has been raised from additional taxes on cigarettes to create a fund for supplying 43 essential drugs free of charge to children under 5 years of age. Drugstores in the public sector sell essential drugs at lower prices. The Government in Haiti has a similar scheme. It has created a national agency, Agapco, to promote and support community-based pharmacies selling prepackaged generic drugs at fixed prices.

By 1971 Peru had already launched a basic drugs programme, including a list of between 230 and 250 generic products, which all government health services were obliged to adhere to in prescribing. The programme, however, encountered serious difficulties, mainly for economic and social reasons; there was also a need to intensify efforts to convince prescribers of the advantages of basic drugs. Furthermore, it was realized that management and quality control needed to be improved. In 1983, an improved list was developed, subdivided into levels of priority and including information on the drugs, but the same problems as had arisen in the first programme remained. Since 1985 new measures have been adopted to rationalize the production of drugs and encourage the use of essential drugs. They include: a national list of basic and essential drugs (68 products) to be supplied to the public sector, 16 of which are delivered in kits to remote areas; and a new regulatory authority (CONAMAD), which has prohibited some of the obsolete combinations and dangerous products still on the market and established a price control system for essential drugs.

All these fresh initiatives face problems in implementation related to the need for additional resources and to encourage and train prescribers to use drugs more rationally. The economic crisis, which was the reason behind the adoption of these policies in Latin America, adds to the difficulties.

Since 1981, Indonesia and Thailand have rationalized drug supply in the public sector, mainly through the use of an essential drugs list. In Indonesia, the annual per capita spending on drugs is about US$ 2.7, 21% being consumed in hospitals and health care institutions. In Thailand the per capita consumption is US$ 6. In Indonesia a national drug policy was formulated in 1983 with the aims of ensuring the availability of drugs to meet the needs of the population, ensuring rational and efficient use of drugs, and promoting local production. In the two countries, essential drugs for the public sector are mainly produced by government-owned companies (Perum Indofama and DT Kimia Farma in Indonesia and the Government Pharmaceutical Organization in Thailand). Drug cooperative funds (Thailand) and community cooperatives (Indonesia) have been established in the villages in recent years to improve the supply of drugs. In Indonesia since 1986, drugs produced by the government-owned factories have been introduced into the private sector and doctors are encouraged to prescribe them for low-income patients, a group that has increased dramatically in size since the fall in world oil prices. Special prescription pads have been issued for the purpose. Pharmacists can replace prescribed branded drugs by these drugs if the patient cannot afford the branded product and agrees to the substitution. The introduction of these cheaper drugs, as price leaders on the market, has had the effect of lowering prices.

While drugs are more widely available in this group of countries, a lot remains to be done in relation to their use. The situation in these 33 countries is in many cases similar to that in countries in group A. Very few provide objective information on a regular basis to health workers and prescribers about drug characteristics, safety, indications, etc. Thailand is an exception; it regularly distributes a prescriber's journal and a drug bulletin free of charge to all prescribers and other health professionals. In Indonesia, it is proposed that pharmaceutical and therapeutic committees should be established in the main hospitals, to act as focal points for drug information and education. In all countries prescribers still depend almost entirely on the pharmaceutical industry for their information. This situation is aggravated by the fact that there is no continuing education and the curricula of schools of medicine, pharmacy, and nursing do not include the essential drugs concept.

Only Indonesia and Thailand have mechanisms such as post-marketing surveillance and monitoring of adverse reactions. National programmes for monitoring of adverse drug reactions were established in the early 1980s and are based on spontaneous reporting from medical and pharmaceutical professions. They are linked to the WHO Collaborating Centre in Uppsala, Sweden. Through the monitoring programme, it was discovered, for instance, that in Indonesia there is a relatively high incidence of anaphy-lactic shock following the use of parenteral antibiotics.

Most of the countries in this group are at stage 2 in the revised UNIDO classification relating to the production of drugs from pharmaceutical chemicals. Indonesia and Pakistan produce some raw materials. In most cases the national industry is weak. In Central America 70% of drugs are imported, and, of the remaining 30%, 20% are produced by multinational companies and 10% by local producers. In Colombia only 5% of finished products are imported; there are 400 production laboratories in the country, 70 multinational firms producing 90% of the products and 330 local producers the remainder. In Thailand there are nearly 200 en-terprises, 14 owned by multinational companies or joint ventures, two state-owned, and the rest local producers. In Indonesia there are 40 multi-national companies and 247 national pharmaceutical manufacturers of various sizes; 95% of drugs are formulated locally and some raw materials are also produced locally. In the African countries local production is less important; there are few production units in each country. The main characteristics of local production units, both in Africa and in Latin America, are: an inadequate physical infrastructure, poor quality control and manufacturing practices, inefficient production, lack of foreign exchange and of market intelligence, and products that do not meet the needs of the public sector. Most of these countries are promoting local production and, in the face of the predominance of the multinational companies, have sought ways to regulate their subsidiaries and encourage national enterprises through regulations covering the control of transfer-pricing (Colombia), price controls, and the regulation of patents (Colombia, Thailand). In addition, in Thailand all pharmaceuticals on the national list of essential drugs that are manufactured by the Government Pharmaceutical Organization must be purchased directly from it by public hospitals (this represents 8–10% of a total pharmaceutical market worth more than US$ 300 million in 1985). In Indonesia subsidiaries of foreign manufacturers are directed towards the production of new innovative drugs and the introduction of new production technology. The new drugs are protected for a period of three years. National manufacturers are directed towards the production of cheaper branded as well as generic drugs, and government-owned factories towards the production of essential drugs and essential raw materials. This policy is enforced through drug registration and regulation of foreign investment.

In conclusion, these countries have introduced a number of essential components of a national drug policy. They are, however, faced by two main groups of problems.

In the poorest countries, mainly African, as long as economic resources and foreign exchange are scarce and not allocated on a regular basis, the situation is going to be very unstable. Some of these countries have to strengthen the ministry of health's negotiating power vis-à-vis the central banks. In certain cases, drastic decisions will have to be taken about the range and quantity of drugs to be imported into the country if essential drugs are to be made available.

In the richer countries the economic crisis has had a considerable effect on the functioning of the public sector in general. Although rationalization of the drug sector has been attained in many cases, the deficiencies of the public sector in manpower, resources, etc. have a negative impact on rationalization, and on the functioning of the regulatory bodies responsible for providing objective information and for registering new products.

The main issues are:

— how to implement the drug policies aimed at making essential drugs available, in the context of the economic crisis, with scarce financial resources, shortage of foreign exchange, lack of trained personnel, and overworked drug regulatory authorities;

— how to improve the rational use of drugs in both the public and the private sector;

— how to procure drugs more efficiently and, where feasible, strengthen the existing local drug industry to make it more relevant to health needs.

Chapter 7

Group C: Countries with high coverage

Group C is the largest of the four groups, comprising 47 developing countries in which between 60% and 90% of the population have access to essential drugs. Thus, of the total population of 1.7 billion, between 170 million and 680 million have no regular access to essential drugs. The level of economic development of most of these countries is far superior to that of groups A and B. The group includes countries with a per capita gross domestic product ranging from US$ 250 to more than US$ 15 000, the average being US$ 2360.

The group is very diverse, including small island countries (Comoros, Saint Lucia, Vanuatu), oil-producing countries (Saudi Arabia), and very large countries with considerable pharmaceutical markets and manufacturing capacity (Brazil, Islamic Republic of Iran). The health situation reflects the diversity of the countries. Life expectancy at birth is generally over 60 years. Infant mortality rates are below 100 per thousand live births: 18 per 1000 in Costa Rica, 17 in Cuba, 32 in Kuwait, 94 in Lesotho, 53 in Mexico. In terms of mortality and morbidity the small island countries and the African countries present the same picture as group B. The others, which are rapidly industrializing developing countries, have morbidity and mortality patterns characteristic of an epidemiological transition period. Gastro-intestinal and respiratory infections continue to be the leading causes of death, but deaths due to chronic diseases and accidents are increasing.

The health sector in most countries comprises both public health services and a private sector. In Latin America social security institutions cover an important part of the population (44% in Mexico) and generally provide drugs at no additional cost. As a result of the economic crisis, there has been an increase in many countries in use of the public health care system by a part of the population that previously preferred to use private services, thereby adding to the burden on the public health services.

Although 10–30% of the population have no regular access to health services, all have some access to modern drugs, mainly through the private sector. The practice of traditional medicine, which was still very consider-able 50 years ago, has decreased dramatically, except in China, Sri Lanka, and some African countries. Some of the popular medical concepts that have developed in relation to traditional substances are now applied to drugs prescribed by physicians or to over-the-counter drugs purchased for self-medication; hence there is a risk of drug misuse and of neglect of serious medical conditions.

Nearly all the countries have an essential drugs list (Table 28 and Annex 2) for their public sector, which in most cases is used for procurement. It is interesting to note that, while most of the countries have a list and a strong policy commitment, 21% have little or no commitment at all (Table 28). These countries are generally high-income oil-producing countries and, although few data are available, the main problems they face appear to be very much like the problems of the developed countries: overconsumption and irrational use and prescribing of drugs.

Group C can be further divided into two categories of countries: those with an essential drugs programme and those with some elements of a national drugs policy.

Table 28. **Distribution of countries in group C (high coverage) according to selected indicators** [a, b]

Level	Policy (%)	Legisla- tion (%)	Essential drugs list (%)	Procure- ment (%)	Distribu- tion (%)	Cover- age (%)	Quality assur- ance (%)	Informa- tion (%)	Man- power develop- ment (%)	Moni- toring (%)
1	21	7	2	26	9	—	—	26	91	45
2	32	17	36	40	51	—	26	70	7	38
3	38	57	62	34	36	100	53	—	—	10
4	—	10	—	—	—	—	17	—	—	—
Data not available	9	9	—	—	4	—	4	4	2	7

[a] Source: WHO secretariat.

[b] For more information see Annexes 1 and 2.

Countries with an essential drugs programme

In the past few years, countries in this category have planned and implemented essential drugs programmes in the public sector. They are mainly low-income African countries (e.g., Botswana, Comoros, Gambia, Kenya, Lesotho, United Republic of Tanzania) and islands in the Caribbean region (e.g. Grenada, Jamaica, Saint Lucia); they have been or still are receiving considerable foreign aid; they are characterized by fairly good procurement and distribution systems; and they use open tendering systems or negotiated procurement. Although a lack of market intelligence still prevents full rationalization of drug procurement mechanisms, these measures have resulted in substantial savings. Health workers are receiving regular training in the use of drugs.

Kenya is a good example of this category. In the past few years, with the support of WHO, it has introduced an essential drugs programme for the rural areas with a limited list of drugs, quantification of drug needs, and drugs packed in kits. This efficient system is now being established at district hospital level. The United Republic of Tanzania is another example, but there the system is totally dependent on foreign support, which raises the question of the sustainability of such schemes in low-income countries. In Gambia also, the procurement and distribution of drugs have been improved dramatically in the past 5–8 years, with a general improvement in the other components of the national drug policy. New legislation has been developed and the drug registration system is being computerized.

Small countries in Latin America have been turning their attention to subregional schemes for joint procurement and quality control. The Eastern Caribbean Drug Service, for instance, collates country forecasts, invites tenders, and through a representative committee awards regional price contracts. For the term of the contract, the agreed supplier is then the sole supplier to the participating countries of each item on the tender. A Caribbean Regional Drug Testing Laboratory has been set up by 14 countries of the region to perform pharmaceutical tests on drugs submitted by any participating government, to investigate specific issues, and to coordinate and support drug control activities in the region.

In many of these countries, however, not all of the elements of a comprehensive drug quality assurance system (including appropriate legislation, inspection, and adequate laboratory services) are in place. Drug registration has only recently been introduced, and inspection and quality control are poorly enforced owing to lack of trained manpower and inadequate facilities and financial resources.

Drug policy is well defined for the public sector, but the private sector is less regulated. This sector is dominated by the multinational companies; 75–80% of drugs, in terms of value, are branded products imported as finished products, and they very often do not meet priority health needs, use up scarce foreign exchange, and are sold at high prices. In 1982, following debates in the Kenyan Parliament on the alleged practice of certain foreign companies of dumping low quality drugs, Kenya adopted a new drug registration scheme and carried out a review that has resulted in a decrease in the number of drugs on the market.

Countries with some elements of a national drug policy

A second category in this group consists of countries that have in place some components of a national drug policy, such as a regulatory administration, quality control laboratories, and an essential drugs list for the public sector (the first list in Sri Lanka dates from 1959, in Chile from 1965, in Brazil from 1972, and in Algeria from 1979). Some of these countries have tried in the past to implement a comprehensive essential drugs policy, but they have encountered major internal and external resistance and have not totally succeeded. Under the pressure of the economic crisis, and influenced by the essential drugs concept, some new initiatives have arisen which aim to increase the availability of drugs to the general public. In Sri Lanka, where the national drug policy dates from 1958, a national seminar on drug policies and management was held in 1985 under the auspices of WHO. The essential drugs list was reviewed and plans were drawn up for introducing a system for quantifying requirements for pharmaceuticals based on standard treatments, and for instituting training and continuing education. In Algeria, the essential drugs list was revised in 1986, a guide on drug use for doctors was prepared, and procurement will be in terms of the products in the list.

Argentina has drawn up a list of 300 single drugs which must be used in the state health services. This has created problems with the national pharmaceutical industry, which mainly produces combination drugs and is afraid of being excluded from the public sector market. To cover the needs of the poorest part of the population, the Government recently created an essential drugs programme, Fondo de Assistencia de Medicamentos (FAM), the resources for which will come from taxes on cigarettes and pharmaceutical specialities. However, this programme, which aims to make available 43 essential drugs to poor families, is encountering various serious problems, such as administrative bottlenecks and legal challenges.

In 1971 Brazil created a state-owned enterprise, Central de Medicamentos (CEME), to rationalize the procurement of medicines for public hospitals and clinics and provide free prescription drugs to the poorest in the population. The first essential drugs list was issued in 1972. The present list contains 231 products, having been reduced in 1987 to counteract the effects of pharmaceutical shortages that arose during 1986 and to ensure adequate supplies. The criteria used for the revision included cost of manufacture, extent of use, and degree to which the raw materials used were locally produced. A further measure to improve supply was the setting up of 19 200 basic pharmacies operating in public health service outlets. Each pharmacy will be supplied with 30 essential drugs in 44 presentations. CEME, which currently serves about six million people, hopes to extend pharmaceutical supplies to the entire needy population, estimated at

50 million people; this will be done by supplying a basic list of about 40 drugs. The second field of activities of CEME is promotion, research, and production of essential drugs. Of the total consumption of drugs in the country, the government health services account for 15%, supplied by publicly owned manufacturing companies.

In Venezuela until recently resources were not too scarce and no real effort was made to rationalize drug policy. Under the effect of the recession, and also because of the influence of the essential drugs concept, Venezuela has set up a commission to investigate ways of producing and distributing the most widely used drugs as generics.

Most of the countries in this category, with the exception of Algeria and Cuba, have a substantial private market with a large number of branded products (24 000 in Brazil), some of which are of doubtful efficacy and many far from meeting the health needs of the population. There is a high consumption of cough remedies, vitamins, and laxatives. National and international consumer movements are active in many of these countries. Recently independent observers have stated that the industry has improved some of its practices. The governments have initiated measures to tighten up drug regulation by more controls on new drug registration and systematic review of existing products. In Latin America, Chile is the only exception to this trend. In that country the marketing of new drugs has been easier since 1973 and the national formulary committee has been abolished. Chile is also the only Latin American country with no price control. However, because of the importance of the market share (35%) of one of the publicly owned laboratories, Laboratorio Chile, which produces and sells cheap generics, the prices of other drugs are aligned with its prices and are thus at a reasonable level.

Despite improvements in legislation, use of drugs is still of concern; not only is there self-medication with prescription drugs but studies have shown the importance of improving prescribing by medical personnel. There is a need for objective information to be supplied to the medical profession to facilitate rational use of drugs in the public and private sector. Although all these countries have a long tradition of drug regulation (Venezuela has rigorous criteria for drug registration that have been copied by other American countries) and quality control, better coordination could improve use of existing resources. Manpower is also an increasing problem in Latin America because of the low salaries in the public sector.

Most of the countries in this category produce finished products and a range of raw materials. As the situation in Mexico is fairly typical of the group and will be described in more detail, no long description will be given here, but it is worth noting that in nearly all the countries reviewed, with the exception of Cuba, Egypt and the Islamic Republic of Iran, the drug supply is mainly in the hands of private industry. Multinational companies have an overwhelming share of the market (with the exception of Argentina, where national producers control 45–50% of the total internal market for finished products). National producers face constraints such as the unavailability or high price of imported raw materials and difficulty in obtaining foreign technology on suitable terms. In order to promote local production countries have developed different approaches. One is the nationalization of foreign subsidiaries, as in Egypt and the Islamic Republic of Iran (page 91). Another is the implementation of selective measures to regulate foreign companies and stimulate growth of domestic enterprises. They include: control of the cost of imports (e.g., by monitoring imports of raw materials through negociations with the pharmaceutical industry, Argentina has been able to save substantial amounts of foreign exchange); joint projects between countries to reduce technological dependence on the multinational companies through promotion of the production of pharma-ceutical chemicals (such a project is under study between Argentina, Brazil, Mexico, and Spain); and elimination of patent protection in order to increase the competitiveness of domestic companies. This elimination of patent protection has led to increased external bilateral and multilateral pressure on the governments concerned and danger of commercial and financial reprisals.

Three countries in this category will be described in more detail. One, Mexico, is quite representative of the group. The other two, China and the Islamic Republic of Iran, have developed successful strategies similar to those already used in Cuba and in Egypt.

Mexico

In Mexico three types of medical institution provide services to the population: institutions serving the general population (which cover 10% of the population); social security institutions (which cover 45% of the population); and the private sector. In 1985 it was estimated that about 13 million people in Mexico had no access to health services of any type; this figure can be expected at least to remain the same if not to increase in the future because of a decrease in resources. Nevertheless, the Ministry of Health is committed to increasing the coverage.

Per capita expenditure on pharmaceuticals has also decreased, from US$ 17.95 in 1982 to US$ 10 in 1983, again owing to the lower purchasing power of the population. Systemic antibiotics are the most widely sold drugs; in 1984 they accounted for 19% of total market sales. Within this class the largest subclass was ampicillin, which accounted for 28% of sales of the class. Vitamins, cough and cold preparations, analgesics, and antirheu-matics each accounted for 5% of sales. Self-medication is widespread in Mexico.

Almost all the drugs consumed are manufactured locally, only 2–3% being imported. Reliance on imported raw materials is, however, high. In 1985, Mexico met about 50% of its needs for raw materials by domestic manufacture.

Multinational companies predominate. However, from 1982 to 1985 Mexican firms increased their share of the market from 28% to 38%, and 16 of them, as against 11 in the past, are among the leading 50 companies. In 1982 the public sector accounted for 25% of sales, the private sector for the remaining 75%. By 1985 sales to the public sector had increased to 40% of the total. In 1984, for the first time, the total sales of Mexican companies to the public sector exceeded those of the multinationals, with 53% as against 47% (44% and 56% in 1982), and a Mexican company now occupies the first place.

The Mexican Government's objectives in the development of its drug policy are in line with those of WHO:

(1) to make good quality essential drugs available to the population at a reasonable price;

(2) to promote the rational use of drugs; and

(3) to promote self-sufficiency and development of the national pharmaceutical industry.

Efforts to this effect have been made over the years. The first list of essential drugs appeared in 1958, the first national drug formulary in 1960, and the national formulary (*Cuadro Básico de Medicamentos*) for drugs in the public sector in 1977. An interministerial commission on the pharmaceutical industry was established in 1977, proposed a set of minimum standards for the facilities and equipment of the drug industry, and consolidated tendering for the procurement of drugs by the health sector. This became official practice in 1980.

Nevertheless, the shortage of drugs experienced in 1982 revealed the structural weaknesses of the drug industry in the country. There was heavy dependence on foreign imports of basic intermediates; dependence also on the multinational companies; difficulty in obtaining appropriate technology; and lack of coordination in research and development. As a result, the Ministry of Health and other bodies concerned implemented an emergency plan to deal with the shortages. Legislation was enacted to control and rationalize the use of drugs and vaccines.

An integrated programme for the development of the pharmaceutical industry was drawn up with the following objectives:

(1) to develop a rational scheme for the production and marketing of drugs satisfying the health needs of the population;

(2) to rationalize the drug market;

(3) to strengthen economic independence by increasing local manufacture of raw materials, to save foreign exchange through the substitution of locally manufactured drugs for imports, and to promote exports;

(4) to establish a solid technological structure as a base for independent development;

(5) to establish a policy of equal prices for equal products; and

(6) to develop a solid local managerial capability based on efficiency, creativity, and innovation.

Legislation and decrees were promulgated to implement the policy. Outside opposition was strong and was mainly directed at the use of generic names without registered trademarks on all products sold to the health sector, the addition of generic names to registered trademarks in the private sector, the elimination of drugs from the register, and the ban on irrational combinations of drugs. In 1984, the Mexican Government decided to change these regulations, and in April 1985 a new set of rules for implementation of the decrees replaced the previous ones.

In the implementation of the new policies, the registration procedure has been modernized and computerized. All the drugs on the drug registry will be reviewed. In the private sector, there are 7000 products representing 950 active ingredients and 3400 combinations, of which 1800 have been classified as irrational. In the past two years 400 of these drugs have been reformulated. In 1987, 51.5% of the drugs in the private sector were single entities (6% being sold under generic name) and 48.5% combination drugs; 27% still need reformulation. Currently, combination drugs are being tackled by the Ministry of Health in its campaign to promote the rational use of drugs in the private sector. The quality control of both the manufacturing process and the products will be improved, good manufacturing practices will be enforced, and a Mexican pharmacopoeia will be published.

The 1976 patent law was modified in 1986. The new law gives process patent protection for pharmaceuticals produced through industrial processes. However, drugs produced through biotechnological processes will not be covered by process patents for 10 years after the amendments come into force. Product protection will be given to the chemicopharmaceutical industry and the biotechnology industry for the next 10 years. For both process and product patents the period of protection will be 14 years. There have been arguments about the impact of these changes on the industry. The multinational companies maintain that the introduction of product patents will benefit the whole industry, while national companies say they are not ready for such a change and that the Government should wait until they have further developed their own industry.

A national formulary for drugs and other inputs to the health sector was prepared and a commission for the revision of the national formulary was established in 1983. A manual on the utilization of the drugs in the national formulary was prepared for health workers.

The procurement scheme for the public sector has been modified to make it more efficient and to create incentives for national producers. Under the new scheme the Government does not have to pick the company making the lowest bid but can choose one that bids within 15% of the lowest price if certain conditions are met. These conditions relate to performance in fulfilling previous orders, investment in manufacture of raw materials, Mexican share of capital, trade balance, and amount of locally manufactured ingredients.

An adverse drug reaction information system was created in 1986.

A programme of free distribution of 60 essential drugs to the poor was instituted in 1987. These drugs may also be retailed at preferential prices.

In conclusion, Mexico, like many other countries that are having to adjust to the economic crisis, has developed a strategy aimed at:

— strengthening its essential drugs policy by improvement of the national formulary, review of the drugs on the market, promotion of rational drug use in the public and private sector, rationalization of procurement, and increased coverage and distribution of drugs to the poor; and

— fostering the development of the national drug manufacturing industry.

The new policies have contributed to improved coverage of the population and to changes in pharmaceutical market structure, in which Mexican firms have traditionally had a small share; the public sector purchasing policy is in fact responsible for the increased share since Mexican firms are preferred as providers. As many of the measures described have only recently been introduced, it is difficult at present to assess their impact and progress.

Islamic Republic of Iran

The Islamic Republic of Iran produced a new drug policy only one year after the Islamic revolution in 1979. Before that the health and drug situation in the country was similar to that in many developing countries at the same socioeconomic level. The aim of the new drug policy was to secure a reliable provision of low-cost good generic drugs for the whole population, and its major objectives were:

— national self-sufficiency in drug production where economically and technically feasible;

— adoption of a national formulary based on generic drugs; and

— development of a coherent government distribution system throughout the country.

While the new drug policy was in most respects in line with the policies recommended by WHO, it was drafted without any outside assistance. First an Iranian national formulary was drawn up, based on generic drugs plus a few branded products where generics were not available. The formulary contained 600 products and 1000 dosage forms, as against some 4000 branded drugs previously on sale. Then a planned system of local production and distribution was developed.

A nationalization law was promulgated in 1980. Foreign pharmaceutical companies all accepted nationalization. A government drug distribution system was established. Quality control was given top priority; all companies have to comply with WHO's Good Manufacturing Practices and British and American standards. Pharmacopoeia standards were adopted for the country and rigorous quality control requirements instituted. The National Food and Drug Laboratory is responsible for drug quality control. In addition, all producers have their own quality control facilities to test the quality of the raw materials, products being processed, and finished products.

The resistance to the new drug policy was strong in the early years, especially from the pharmaceutical companies. This prolonged negotiations. Moreover, some physicians and patients opposed the new policy because of the fewer drugs available and of the requirement for generic prescribing. Little international attention was given to the changes.

After nationalization, many multinational companies were not prepared to supply essential raw materials, or demanded prices for them that were considered unacceptably high. The raw materials bought by the Government from other sources often proved to be unreliable. The resistance has now decreased and almost all imported raw materials and finished products are bought from well known manufacturers in western Europe and Japan. Thus, the Government has been able to achieve most of its objectives.

Before the revolution, 75% of the 4000 branded products were imported and the remainder produced locally by 42 companies, mainly subsidiaries and licensees of multinational companies; only a few were national. In 1985, 80% of the value and 90% of the volume of the pharmaceuticals distributed were produced locally. The pharmaceutical industry is largely government-controlled, being either government-owned or under government supervision. The companies under supervision are mainly multinational companies that were nationalized, and they account today for approximately 70% of national production. About 3% of the market is supplied by private companies. The drugs manufactured are mainly generic, as a result of which approximately 70% of all prescriptions now use generic names.

The Iranian pharmaceutical industry still depends on imports of raw materials. Annual planning of pharmaceutical production is carried out by the Office of Pharmaceuticals and Medical Equipment of the Ministry of Health, the estimates of quantity being related to local production capacity; production quotas are agreed with firms and excess requirements are met by imports. The local producers state their needs for raw materials and the office considers the requests. Procurement is handled directly by the manufacturers, but prices and quality are closely supervised by the office, which also coordinates orders to obtain the maximum bulk discount and establishes a foreign exchange budget in collaboration with the Central Bank. These procedures enable the Iranian drug supply system to manage procurement and production efficiently and to obtain extremely competitive prices while maintaining high quality.

Imports of finished products are handled by the Iranian Pharmaceutical Institute and by some of the larger distributors. The import prices of finished products are comparable with prices obtained by other countries, WHO, and UNICEF in the international generic market.

Previously, drug distribution was left to the market. The new government system consists of eleven distributors who handle all distribution to both the public and the private sector. They have a countrywide network of depots and computerized information systems providing data on orders, deliveries, and stocks. Distribution is planned on the basis of a detailed statement of the drug quantities to be distributed to each area, agency, and institution, the statement being prepared on consumption estimates within the local budgets. The prices of locally manufactured pharmaceuticals and medical supplies are fixed by the office and reviewed once a year. Drug prices have in fact not increased for several years, and those in 1986, after allowing for inflation, were about 25% lower in real terms than they were in 1983.

The Islamic Republic of Iran has a high level of drug consumption, estimated in 1985 to be US$ 25 per capita, the highest in the WHO Eastern Mediterranean Region. Many prescription drugs are also available as over-the-counter drugs, and people often buy them as a way of avoiding medical consultation fees. Of this consumption 30% in terms of value are anti-infective drugs, and 10% are analgesics. Polypharmacy is still common in the country; prescriptions normally have 3 or 4 items and up to 6 is not unusual. More than 70% of all the medicines prescribed are generic. So far, implementation of the new drug policy has not had a great impact on the consumption pattern, apart from increasing generic prescribing.

Before the revolution drug information was mainly provided by 3000 medical representatives from the pharmaceutical companies whose drugs were distributed. Drug information is now the responsibility of the Government. The six state-controlled distribution centres are staffed by doctors and pharmacists who are responsible for providing the health staff with information. For this purpose 1.5% of the revenue from each distributing centre's total sales has been allocated for the provision of information. The Ministry of Health provides up-to-date information through government-published journals containing articles translated from other journals and also a regularly updated list of approved drugs.

At this early stage it would appear that the drug policy introduced by the Islamic Republic of Iran has improved self-sufficiency, drug quality control, distribution, and access to essential drugs. As in most countries, however, the use of drugs could be greatly rationalized.

China

Since the founding of the People's Republic of China in 1949 the Government has given considerable attention to the health of the population. The general indicators show that the health standards of the country already approach those of developed countries. The average life expectancy of the population rose from a pre-1949 level of 35.6 years to 67.9 years in 1984. The pre-1949 birth rate of 35 per 1000 fell to 17.5 per 1000 by 1984, the death rate of 25.0 per 1000 to 6.7. Infections and parasitic diseases have more or less been replaced by cerebrovascular disease, heart disease, and cancer as the main causes of death.

Four basic principles were adopted by the 1950 National Health Congress in order to increase and improve the health services provided at all levels of the society. These principles were:

— to orient health care services towards the needs of workers, peasants, and the military;

— to place emphasis on preventive medicine;

— to unite practitioners of traditional Chinese medicine and "Western" medicine;

— to promote the participation of the population in health care.

In the past few years several steps have been taken towards the development of the health system. Health legislation has been strengthened and a number of provisions governing administration, regulations, and standards have been revised. Disease eradication programmes, such as mass treatment, have been instituted. Attention has been given to occupational health, food hygiene, and school health. Family planning is given high priority in all health programmes.

Free medical services are available to students and government officials and employees, who number approximately 110 million people or 11% of the population. Health care coverage is also provided for their families. A number of services are free of charge for the general population, such as provision of contraceptives, immunization, and chemoprophylaxis. In addition, insurance-covered plans exist for workers within the services and industries under government control. Various forms of optional medical insurance are also available. The self-employed do not have free or insurance-covered medical care but have to pay a small fee.

Traditional Chinese medicine is an important part of the health system in China. It has a long and strong tradition, of which the earliest national pharmacopoeia in the world, listing 850 different herbs, forms part. It is oriented towards treating the whole body, paying special attention to the development of illness and the interaction between the patient and the environment. The Chinese Government has taken great care to develop traditional medicine and to integrate it with Western medicine; today, it has equal status with Western medicine, and is included in the Government's health policy. The State Administration of Traditional Chinese Medicine is responsible for it and legislation was recently drafted for the purpose of speeding up its development. Traditional treatment is regarded as safe, acceptable, and effective for common everyday illnesses and is available at low cost.

The main objectives of the Government have been to meet the priority needs of the population through local production and to develop the country's export potential. Major problems encountered were related to the need to improve quality control, to increase research, and to strengthen international marketing capacity. Today China is 90% self-sufficient. In the 1950s priority in production was given to bulk antibiotics, sulfonamides, antipyretics, vitamins, and drugs for endemic disease and tuberculosis. In the 1960s production was expanded to include steroids, anticancer agents, drugs for cardiovascular diseases, products for upper respiratory tract infections and asthma, and X-ray contrast media. In 1985 the pharmaceutical chemical industry output of 58 million kg covered 1400 different substances.

Approximately 1833 manufacturers are engaged in pharmaceutical production, of which 478 produce traditional Chinese medicines.

In 1986 the value of Western medicines rose to 12 600 million yuan (US$ 3000 million), an increase of 17.5% from 1985. The value of traditional medicines was 2500 million yuan (an 8.6% increase).

China's National Import and Export Corporation of Medicine and Health Care Products is the body responsible for the import and export of medical supplies of drugs and instruments. The Corporation is under the control of the Ministry of Foreign Trade. It distributes imported goods either directly to special purchasers or to the national distribution network. Importation of drugs is regulated by law and restricted to small quantities of drugs that are difficult to produce and specialized products for which no production plant exists in the country. In spite of this, imports increased more than tenfold in the period 1970–85, but at the same time remained a small percentage of total imports. The import of pharmaceutical items has changed from mainly finished products (62% of the total in 1981) to raw materials.

China is a major international supplier of pharmaceutical chemicals and also one of the largest producers of antibiotics, vitamins, and sulfonamides. It exports approximately 40% by weight (23 million kg) of all bulk pharmaceutical chemicals produced. This, however, amounts to only 7% of the yuan value of annual sales. In 1986 exports of pharmaceuticals and traditional Chinese medicines were worth US$ 600 million, an increase of 17% over 1985. In 1985 the increase was 11.5% over 1984. Overall, China has a strong favourable trade balance for health care products, of US$ 200–300 million a year. In 1986, excluding medical instruments (which are mainly imported), the excess was estimated at US$ 500 million. Traditional Chinese medicines account in value for approximately 60% of exports.

The major export items are bulk tetracycline, lincomycin, chloramphenicol, and heparin. In addition, bulk steroids (basic materials), dexamethasone, and triamcinolone are manufactured for export on a large scale.

To strengthen the pharmaceutical industry further, the Government has decided to introduce good manufacturing practices to meet internationally acceptable standards; to develop the production of special high-value exports and sophisticated items; and to develop traditional Chinese medicines in Western-style formulations, or the active ingredients isolated from the medicines and chemical modifications of the ingredients. For this purpose China is seeking foreign support and international collaboration and actively promoting international contacts. The previous restrictive trade policy has been modified and more favourable tax laws have been introduced to attract foreign investment. A number of joint-venture contracts of twenty years' duration have been completed with 50:50 capital participation. In 1986 two had already started production.

Within the country the National Corporation of Pharmaceutical Distribution is responsible for the procurement and supply of all pharmaceutical chemicals and medicines. The distribution is carried out through a network of distribution centres throughout the country. There are six national stations for medical procurement and supply. In addition, in 1985 there were 2600 wholesale units and 50 000 retail outlets scattered through the country. About 90% in value of all medical supplies are supplied by wholesalers to hospitals, and less than 10% are sold at low prices through retail units.

A national essential drugs list of 278 products was established as a result of a campaign started in 1979, and in 1984 a manual on their use was published and distributed.

A major part of traditional Chinese medicines are distributed directly to the population through traditional Chinese pharmacies. Such medicines (brands and herbals) represent about 40% of domestic sales (Table 29). In urban areas they are mainly sold through pharmacies, but in rural parts through a variety of outlets. In 1984, there were approximately 147 500 traditional druggists. The practitioners work within the traditional Chinese pharmacies and are an important component of health care.

Table 29. **Value of domestic market sales in China, 1980–85**[a]

Year	Western products (millions of yuan)	Traditional Chinese products	
		Brands (millions of yuan)	Herbals (millions of yuan)
1980	3273	1043	1417
1981	3737	1273	1486
1982	5094	1531	1589
1983	5653	1817	1825
1984	5922	2017	2032
1985	6126	2298	2066

[a] Source: *Pharmaceutical business opportunities with China – an analysis.* Richmond, Surrey, SCRIP, 1987.

Quality control institutes have been established in all the provinces and in most prefectures and municipalities. The Chinese authorities continue to improve their quality control methods, a process that began with the Drug Control Act, 1984, and is partly aimed at increasing the industry's exports by meeting international standards for testing and production.

The annual per capita consumption of drugs in 1985 was US$ 4.94. However, the price of drugs in China is much lower than in other countries. There is no doubt that the population has benefited from the boom in pharmaceutical production and now has access to a much wider range of drugs, including sophisticated drugs. Despite this, the health care system has encountered drug shortages. A survey of hospitals and drug stores in Beijing, published in the Chinese newspaper the *Guangming Daily* in early 1987, revealed that the Beijing Pharmaceutical Company, which supplies about 1500 different medicines to over 200 hospitals and drug stores, could meet only 65–70% of its monthly orders. The reasons alleged were lack of communication between manufacturer, distributor, and purchaser; closure of some factories that did not meet the required standards of hygiene and safety; and concentration of companies on more commercial lines and cosmetics instead of essential drugs.

In the future China is expected to expand and develop further pharmaceutical production for the international as well as the domestic market.

The objectives of the seventh five-year plan (1986–1990) include: availability of drugs to meet the needs of the people; improvements in production; research on and development of new drugs; priority for biotechology; development of effective new drugs, biochemical diagnostic reagents, immunological drugs, and bioengineering technologies; and the development of other traditional health-promoting agents. Efforts are being made to strengthen research and development; for this purpose a national institute of pharmaceutical research and development is projected and is expected to be established in 1988. It will include the Institute of Pharmaceuticals, the Institute of Traditional Drugs, and the Institute of Biotechnology. The institute will be concerned with coordinating and organizing national pharmaceutical research and development and undertaking major pharmaceutical research projects. International firms will be able to participate in joint research. Biotechnology is given top priority in the science and technology development programmes.

In this third group the policy and experience of China and the Islamic Republic of Iran stand out. The changes made in the health and pharmaceutical sector and the improvements in health conditions achieved have come about in the context of broad-based social change and transformation of the entire system. Other countries have also made efforts to implement rational drug policies; these efforts are generally too recent for their impact to be assessed, but it is already apparent that internal constraints (lack of expertise, of information, and of enforcement measures), external pressures, and weak political commitment may in many cases slow down implementation. The main issues for countries in group C can be summarized as follows: how to secure the supply of raw materials, to improve the coverage of the poorest people in the population, and to improve the rational use of drugs in the public and the private sectors.

Chapter 8

Group D: Developed countries

Group D comprises the developed countries. Many aspects of the situation in this group have been described in Part I of this report, such as the increasing activity of generic producers, mainly in the United States of America, the role of the research-based companies and changes in their strategies, the structure of drug consumption, and the problems linked with the use of drugs. Therefore this chapter will concentrate on the major trends and issues.

The indicators used for groups A, B, and C are not specific enough to be applied to the developed countries. Essential drugs lists are not generally used there. There are, however, notable exceptions, for example the drugs that can be prescribed by general practitioners in the National Health Service in the United Kingdom and the hospital formularies in many public and private hospitals in several countries. The availability of drugs is assured in most developed countries, and quality control systems and drug regulatory arrangements function properly. The past decade has been characterized by the strengthening of the drug regulatory agencies, the promotion of information for health care providers and the public, and the development of post-marketing surveillance and systems for reporting adverse drug reactions. The need clause, i.e., a clause restricting registration of drugs to those for which there is a definite medical need, used in Norway (12) has been a subject of considerable discussion in international gatherings and elsewhere; although it has not been adopted by other countries, it has led to questions about the comparative efficacy of drugs. Efforts to speed up registration and decrease drug lag have been made in the USA. In the European Region, harmonization of drug registration has been pursued in the light of the plans to abolish trade barriers in the internal market in 1992. The outcome is not yet clear; possibilities range from mutual recognition of individual authorities to the creation of a supranational body. Two important events in 1986 were the introduction of a drug export bill in the USA and a resolution of the European Parliament on drug exports. The first authorized, under certain conditions, the export of drugs not approved in the USA to certain countries considered to have a well developed drug regulatory authority. However, drugs that have been disapproved or for which approval has been withdrawn, or that are otherwise restricted for safety reasons, may not be exported. The second called for a directive that medicines banned in the European Economic Community or whose use is restricted should not be exported unless authorities in the importing country specifically request them; further action has now to be decided on by the European Commission.

Although the situation in the developed countries has improved, many problems remain in relation to the rational use of drugs. To judge by the large number of publications dealing with the subjects, polypharmacy, irrational prescribing, and lack of compliance are still common in all developed countries. Governments are becoming more and more involved in trying to improve the quality of prescribing. The most widely used approach is to furnish impartial data on drugs to physicians; official publications exist in almost all countries that provide therapeutic advice to help prescribers, for example the *British National Formulary* in the United Kingdom, the *Fiches de transparence* in France, *Kompas* in the Netherlands, and the *Physicians' Desk Reference* in the United States of America. Private publications in the health field without drug advertisements are also to be found in larger numbers than a few years ago. Information alone has been shown to be insufficient to improve prescribing practices radically. Other methods are used: the monitoring of doctors by committees, the review of prescriptions by a peer group, the feedback of information about the doctors' prescribing, the restriction of advertisements, and the placing of limits on prescription of certain drugs. Experimental methods have also been tested; in the United Kingdom, for instance, government officials trained in the selling techniques of the pharmaceutical industry visit practitioners to encourage generic prescribing and promote reliance on academic sources of information.

These efforts to improve prescribing are closely linked with efforts to contain expenditure on drugs; indeed, a main concern of governments in developed countries is the increase in expenditure on health care and drugs. In most cases, with the exception of the USA, the health care system is not funded directly by the patient but by government and/or insurance companies. The systems have shown a steady growth in cost and account for an increasing proportion of the gross domestic product. Governments are therefore trying to control the growth; nearly all countries have adopted methods for controlling the cost of pharmaceutical prescriptions. The methods are diverse, ranging from reducing the price of drugs to attempting to influence prescribing and demand.

Direct control of the price of pharmaceuticals has been the most common method in the past ten years in certain countries (e.g., France and Spain) and partly explains the wide differences in the prices charged for drugs between European countries. In 1986, on the basis of a relative price index, prices in Spain were 100, in France 113, in the United Kingdom 200, in the Netherlands 230, and in the Federal Republic of Germany 251 (67). Direct control is strongly opposed by the research-based pharmaceutical industry on the grounds that it endangers its financial situation and therefore its research potential. Control has often been dropped by governments advocating free enterprise; in addition, it has not succeeded in reducing the total cost of drugs, since prices have remained stable but consumption has increased.

In the last few years, attempts to influence prescribing and demand have been more popular. They have included limitation of the number of pharmaceutical products that will be reimbursed by the health insurance scheme, as in the United Kingdom, where a number of products, while still prescribable, are not reimbursable. Through this measure, according to the Department of Health and Social Security, the Government saved £75 million in the first year. The list seems to have had the added effect of making doctors more aware of generic drugs. Although no precise data are available, some patients probably shifted partly to over-the-counter drugs. The Federal Republic of Germany introduced a list of self-limiting disorders; the cost of drugs prescribed for these disorders is not reimbursed.

Similar measures have been taken by Denmark, the Netherlands, and other countries. Although the measures are too recent to have been fully evaluated, some problems are already appearing that reduce their effect, notably a substantial shift from low-cost items that are not permitted to high-cost items that are on the permitted list.

The second measure taken by governments is increased cost-sharing by the consumer. In Sweden, patients now have to pay the first SKr 60 (US$ 9) of any prescription; only above this level does the health insurance pay. Furthermore, a number of cough suppressants and expectorants are no longer reimbursable. In France, different categories of drugs have different cost-sharing rates. Drugs specific for a limited list of diseases are paid for in full by the social security; for other diseases the patient pays 10%, 40%, or 60% of the cost and the last category has recently been enlarged to decrease the cost to social security. Prescription charges were introduced in Norway in 1980 and in the Netherlands in 1983, and they were raised in the Federal Republic of Germany in 1983. In Japan, where drugs accounted for 30% of total spending on health care in 1985, the Government has tried to slow down consumption by cuts in reimbursement.

Other measures include constraints on prescribing and dispensing. In Norway, doctors must prescribe the cheapest product when initiating treatment for 35 chronic diseases. The main requirement is that a generic rather than a branded drug should be prescribed and dispensed. There is little experience of drug substitution and generic prescribing in Europe, although there is now a tendency to encourage generic prescribing, for instance in Sweden. In Canada and the USA drug substitution is increasing when multiple-source drug products are prescribed. All the states of the USA have abolished antisubstitution laws and have explicitly authorized product substitution by the pharmacist; however, the laws differ from state to state. In most, pharmacists are permitted to substitute unless the physician has indicated otherwise on the prescription form. In some, substitution is compulsory. In 1985, pharmacists substituted generics in 35% of prescriptions written for branded products (36). As the patents of more brand drugs expire, more alternatives will become available and the saving in cost for consumers is likely to be significant.

Doctors do not seem particularly opposed to the substitution of generics for branded drugs. According to a study in Canada, only one prescription in 120 in the province of Manitoba bears the instruction "Do not substitute". The figure is one in 200 in Ontario against one in 20 in the USA (*68*). In fact, the main factor leading to the use of brand names is that it is easier, since brand names are short and catchy; prescribers are often not aware of the cost of branded drugs, so do not take it into account in making the decision to prescribe.

Substitution is encouraged by the Government of the United States of America. A book entitled *Approved drug products with therapeutic equivalence evaluation* was issued in 1980 by the Food and Drug Administration to aid pharmacists in selecting drug substitutes. The 1987 edition contains more than 9000 ethical drug products, with a coding system indicating whether the products are equivalent or not suitable for substitution.

Generic prescribing is less common, but studies show that it is increasing; generic names were used in about 19% of entries on drugs in patient records collected as part of a year-long sample of American office-based physicians in 1985. There was at the same time a substantial decline in the proportion of combination drugs, from 26% in 1981 to 20% in 1985 (*69*).

The wide acceptance of these two concepts in the USA is mainly due to pressure from consumers. Unlike European countries, government health care coverage in the USA is limited to the poor and to certain categories of the population, the two existing programmes, Medicare and Medicaid, at present covering 50 million people. Insurance systems exist, but the consumer pays more than 50% of drug costs out of his or her own pocket.

The measures described have generally been accompanied by other measures such as:

— the introduction of a list of prices in the national formulary (United Kingdom);

— an increased use of drug formularies in hospitals and the creation of hospital formulary committees;

— feedback to doctors on their prescribing habits to encourage economic prescribing (France);

— the imposition of penalties on physicians for heavy prescribing (United Kingdom);

— the dissemination of guidelines on dispensing (France).

The main consequence of these measures in European countries has been a shift from public to private spending, a shift that is encouraged by governments to limit public expenditure and increase self-medication.

Self-medication has always been a common method of treating temporary health problems; until the 1930s non-prescription drugs accounted for the large majority of pharmaceutical sales. With the development of national health insurance schemes and the evolution of professional medical services, much larger sections of the population had access to prescribed drugs, and over-the-counter drug sales dropped. In France in 1970, 24% of all the drugs sold were non-prescription drugs; in 1980 the proportion was 12%. With the various cost-containment measures the trend has been reversed in recent years. There are other reasons for the increase in self-medication: awareness of the limits of modern medicine; recognition by the individual of responsibility for his or her own health; and the trend towards reviewing certain medicinal products available only on prescription to determine whether they should not be released for use in self-treatment (as for example the release of ibuprofen as an analgesic with dose limitation in Japan, the Netherlands, the United Kingdom, and the United States of America). Other active substances released from prescription in certain countries are hydrocortisone (for topical use), oral loperamide, econazole, miconazole, tioconazole, and terfenadine maleate. In 1985 in the USA the releases from prescription meant that 150 million fewer prescriptions were written (70). In France the Government seeks to encourage self-medication by simplifying registration procedures for over-the-counter drugs.

This trend reveals a change in attitude. The late 1970s were the years of "rational" drugs; in the late 1980s, under the pressure of the economic crisis and the trend towards free enterprise, governments and a sizeable proportion of the general public seem to accept that it is not always feasible to achieve a scientific solution for therapeutic problems; human beings refuse to be always rational.

In conclusion, the main issue in this group of countries is how to achieve rational and economical prescribing and use of drugs. Governments are mainly concerned with reducing drug costs in the public sector. Although rational prescribing and economical prescribing are often closely linked, there may be a danger in placing the main emphasis on economy; after all, the ultimate objective is health. Apart from problems relating to the effectiveness of cost-control measures, some adverse consequences of some of these measures have already been noted, as for instance a fall in the consumption of essential drugs such as insulin.

The effects of different cost-containment strategies and increased self-medication on health status, expenditure on drugs, and the pharmaceutical industry need to be assessed in the near future to enable governments to draw up rational drug policies reconciling health and economic goals.

103

Chapter 9

Conclusions

The present situation

The grossly unequal distribution of drugs between developed and developing countries has not changed much in the past decade. In 1985, 75% of the world's population still accounted for less than a quarter of total drug consumption, and between 1.3 and 2.5 billion people had little or no regular access to the most essential drugs. This uneven distribution of drug consumption is associated with uneven distribution of drug production, which is still concentrated in a few developed countries. As in the past, large multinational companies play a key role in production and trade, and pharmaceutical innovation continues to make an important contribution to health. Nevertheless, throughout the world, but mainly in the developing countries, there are diseases for which the treatment is inadequate, and new drugs are urgently needed. However, more detailed investigation of this grim picture shows that important changes, which are not always discernible in the global figures, have occured at both the international and the country level.

The past 10–15 years have witnessed a major debate on the question of drugs, a debate kindled by, *inter alia*, the vast number of drugs on the market, increased awareness of the potency of drugs, the cost of drug treatment, the potential for developing new drugs, and the undermedication or overmedication of large segments of the world's population. Increasing attention has been paid by governments to developing mechanisms to improve the availability and rational use of drugs. With the growing awareness of the need for a national drug policy as part of a national health policy, many developed and developing countries, for different reasons, have tried to rationalize their drug sector. Some have drawn up limited lists for general practitioners. Others have embarked on national essential drugs programmes to make better use of the scarce resources available. Although some developing countries have been slow in implementing essential drugs programmes, none has rejected the concept and nearly all have a list of essential drugs under their generic names. It can be assumed that the coverage of the population with essential drugs has increased in the past five years. Consumers have also played an important role in advocating the provision of more and better drug information to the public and in supporting the creation and aims of a national drug policy. The academic world has also been concerned about the irrational use of drugs and has promoted more intensively improvements in the prescribing practices of health practitioners. The concept of rational drug use is gaining greater support and appears on the agenda of most meetings dealing with public health.

Nevertheless, it is evident from this report that the situation still gives cause for concern. Few, if any, countries have attained the objectives of making effective and safe low-cost drugs available to the entire population, ensuring that they are used rationally, and developing technically and financially sound national production of drugs in support of the economic growth and overall development strategy of the country.

Although the situation in individual countries varies enormously, some general conclusions can be drawn about the problems and constraints and the opportunities created by new developments at the international and national level.

National drug policies

It is clear that the first requirement in developing a national drug policy is political commitment. If this commitment is lacking, a rational policy cannot be formulated or, above all, implemented. However, this report has shown that, even when commitment is present, there are many obstacles to the implementation of a national drug policy. Essential drugs policies and programmes have been adopted by more than 40 countries with the objective of making the needed drugs available to the public sector in the right quantities and at affordable prices. In many developed countries, steps have been taken to rationalize the national drug policy. But internal and external pressures, the lack of resources, of a proper infrastructure, and of the manpower required, weakness of the ministries of health, absence of management and planning ability, and the economic crisis all slow down progress. The economic crisis has exacerbated the problem of providing essential drugs by on the one hand decreasing the resources available and on the other increasing the health and other problems of the population.

In some countries the economic crisis has been seen as an opportunity to rationalize the entire system from the importation to the utilization of drugs in order to save money. Moreover, all those concerned — the government, the pharmaceutical industry, consumer groups, health professionals, and the general public — are aware that the use of drugs needs to be, and can be, improved. This awareness is enhanced by the experience gained over the past five years in many countries, and explains the interest of bilateral and multilateral agencies in essential drugs programmes.

It can be expected that in the future yet more countries will develop their own drug programmes and policies and increased attention will be given to the long-term sustainability of the programmes by the countries them-selves, the donor community, and the international organizations through, *inter alia*, cost-recovery schemes and ways and means of obtaining hard currencies. There is also a growing trend for governments in most countries to take an active part in determining the way providers of pharmaceuticals should operate, using a wide range of approaches to develop policies and regulations that benefit the majority of the population. They continue to be opposed by groups with different interests represented in or influencing governments, which lobby against changes that may harm their position. Having raised the alarm in previous years, consumer groups continue to promote public access to more and better information about products, greater availability of drugs for the poorest members of the population, and lower prices.

Double standards in the marketing and promotion of drugs in developing countries have been the subject of wide debate in recent years. WHO has developed ethical criteria[1] for medicinal drug promotion that could be adapted by governments and used by all those concerned. Independent observers have noted an improvement since the introduction of a voluntary code of marketing practices by the International Federation of Pharmaceu-tical Manufacturers Associations (IFPMA). The general trend in dealing with these very sensitive issues is towards responsible cooperation rather than confrontation. The outcome of these conflicts and negociations will, together with political commitment and investment of resources, deter-mine the capacity of countries to attain their health goals.

Drug regulatory authorities

While there is a long tradition of pharmaceutical regulation in developed countries, the past decade has been characterized by the strengthening of the regulatory agencies, the promotion of information, the reporting of adverse drug reactions, and the development of post-marketing surveil-lance. Efforts have also been made to speed up the registration process. Opinions about the future of regulation in developed countries differ. Some think that it will not be very different from what it is today; safety and efficacy will continue to be prerequisites to registration. Others believe that developments in the electronic exchange of information, greater accep-tance of data from other countries, standardized formats for clinical and preclinical studies, and the need for speedier product registration will increase the pressure on regulatory agencies and lead eventually to their worldwide standardization.

---

[1] For further information, write to Action Programme on Essential Drugs, World Health Organization, 1211 Geneva 27, Switzerland.

In developing countries, although only a few drug regulatory authorities are fully functioning, there is a trend towards developing small but effective drug regulatory authorities. In this context the availability of information is crucial. In the past few years, WHO has considerably increased the dissemination of validated information, thus enabling governments to take more rational decisions.

Drug procurement and availability

The same constraints as operate in developing countries in the implementation of a national drug policy operate in attempts to improve the availability of essential drugs. The lack of foreign exchange, the absence of a rational system of procurement with a good selection and quantification of the drugs needed, and the difficulty in obtaining information on suppliers and on prices of finished goods and raw materials are additional problems. However, a large number of countries have achieved some progress in this field by taking advantage of the wide availability of generic drugs at low cost on the international market, regional cooperation, cost-recovery schemes, guidelines for the selection and quantification of drugs, and the services offered by the supply division of UNICEF (UNIPAC) and other non-profit organizations (e.g., IDA, ECHO). As long as rationalization applies to the public sector only, the opposition is not too strong; but the situation is different when it is applied to the private sector, as seen in Bangladesh. Success in the years to come will depend on the capacity of health systems in a period of economic crisis to create efficient, fair, flexible sources of finance ensuring the sustainability of the drug policies and programmes.

In developed countries cost-containment measures in the health sector will no doubt continue. A consequence will be promotion of investment in the production of drugs that will decrease hospitalization, the development of formularies at hospital level and, in some countries, the establishment of limited lists of drugs.

It is forecasted that, by the year 2000, the pharmaceutical market in both developed and developing countries will have increased to at least US$ 200 billion. It is also expected that the current trend towards internationalization of sales and research and development will continue, as well as the tendency to mergers, with the bigger pharmaceutical companies acquiring the smaller ones. Only a few biotechnology firms will have enough capital to develop, register, and market their own products. The generic market, generic prescribing, and drug substitution may also be expected to increase as a result of population increases, efforts to improve the health care coverage in developing countries, and pressures on prices in developed countries. These pressures may also have an impact on research efforts.

Research

Drugs that will be on the market by the 1990s have already been developed; thus current research is on drugs that may be expected to appear in the late 1990s. The five leading categories are expected to be: cardiovascular drugs, antibiotics, psychotherapeutic products, antispasmodics, and drugs to combat cancer. However, the spread of acquired immunodeficiency syndrome (AIDS) will lead many companies to step up research on antiviral products. The effect of AIDS has already been seen on the stock market, with sharp rises in the share prices of companies considered to have a potentially effective treatment.

The emergence of biotechnology could dramatically reverse the decrease in research and development output alleged to have taken place in recent years. The development of monoclonal antibodies, recombinant DNA, genetic engineering, and receptor identification seems likely to have a profound effect on the future of the pharmaceutical industry. The challenge for the biotechnology companies in the next years lies in the commercial-ization of their products, the financing of their enterprise, reasonable patent protection, and the affordability of their products.

The aging of the population in developed countries is also likely to have important repercussions on the pharmaceutical market and on research. New kinds of drugs will be needed to enhance memory and to treat chronic and degenerative diseases, as well as new drug-delivery systems. Ways will have to be developed to encourage investment in the research and development of orphan drugs, i.e., drugs to combat diseases that do not affect large numbers of people. Diseases that affect large segments of the population in developing countries will probably benefit indirectly from these developments. Discussions will continue on how to reconcile the need to encourage research on unsolved health problems with the need to make medicines available at reasonable cost to society.

Production

Some of the larger developing countries have maturing pharmaceutical industries producing bulk materials and finished products covering most domestic needs and increasingly including exports. Many larger countries are nearly self-sufficient in the production of finished drugs but almost completely dependent on imports of bulk raw materials. Many of the least developed countries have a few formulation plants. These plants, with notable exceptions, have been largely unsuccessful in producing drugs at an internationally competitive price; without supporting industries or trained staff, and with difficulty in securing a position in the local market, many operate at low capacity and the added value from the local production of generic drugs is low.

The larger middle-income countries are likely to move towards increased self-reliance at an acceptable cost. It is quite likely that some of the maturing industries will develop innovative drugs as a result of increased investment in research and development. Many smaller countries will need to find internal or external support for the rehabilitation or modernization of their existing formulation plants; otherwise they will be forced to continue subsidizing inefficient production.

Judging from present trends, however, the developing world's share of pharmaceutical production is likely to remain small, although an increasing number of developing countries will manufacture drugs as part of their overall development strategy, to keep costs low and save hard currency. How far they will succeed will depend greatly on the size of the market, their competitiveness, their willingness to seek the technology they need and the conditions of its transfer, local ability to adapt and develop technology, and the commitment of goverments to their support. It will be a challenge for those countries to reconcile economic and health goals in the production of drugs and to ensure the production of low-cost good quality essential drugs.

Some developments in the past few years have created, and will probably continue to create, new opportunities for local production. The patents of a number of products have expired and those of some of the top products in the world market will expire before 1990; there is wider acceptance of generics among the public; technology is increasingly available; market intelligence on raw materials has improved in developing countries; regional cooperation is developing.

It may be expected that the international pharmaceutical industry will try to maintain its position as a producer of drugs in, and exporter of drugs to, developing countries. The question of patents will continue to be debated, and the broader economic and political situation will determine the capacity of developing countries to formulate and manage their own drug policy. International organizations such as UNCTAD, UNIDO, and WHO are taking an increasing part in providing technical support and information to developing countries.

Use of drugs

The procurement or production and distribution of drugs require resources, knowledge, and skills but are fairly mechanical processes that do not call for changes in behaviour. This it not so for the use of drugs, which is a much more complex issue; no country, even the most developed, has totally succeeded in improving the prescribing patterns of medical personnel or the use of drugs by the public. Many obstacles exist to the rational use of drugs, ranging from lack of objective information and of continuing education and training in pharmacology to the methods of promotion employed by the pharmaceutical industry, the shortage of well organized drug regulatory authorities, the presence of large numbers of drugs on the market, excessive demand by the patient, the prevalent belief that "every ill has a pill", and the attitudes of members of the medical profession, who only too often are reluctant to change their practices and view any restriction as a threat to the doctor's freedom to prescribe.

Governments, however, often for cost-containment reasons, have become more aware of the problems linked with irrational consumption and polypharmacy. Some sectors in the academic world have also become conscious of the dangers of insufficient training in pharmacology. Hospital drug committees have been set up, and independent publications discuss the rational use of drugs, including the role of the pharmacist and the ways of increasing it. Consumers are being sensitized to the issue by such publications and by the media. All these new developments present opportunities for improving the situation.

Nevertheless, much more remains to be done. Increased self-medication will require more and better education of both the public and health professionals so as to avoid irrational use of drugs. The danger of drug interactions may also increase and it is expected that adverse reactions will be under-reported since use of over-the-counter drugs may not be reported to or recorded by the doctor. Monitoring of product safety for over-the-counter drugs will probably have to be improved at the level of the pharmacies.

Success in achieving rational use of drugs in the future will depend to a large extent on the ability of governments, WHO, the academic world, health practitioners, the pharmaceutical industry, and consumers to develop information strategies and generate ideas on the most effective role of drugs in society and within the health sector. Given the increased awareness of the problems linked with the use of drugs, current efforts to improve and disseminate the information available, to train health personnel more efficiently, and to educate the public will be intensified. It is certain, however, that the rational use of drugs remains a challenge.

Finally, the essential drugs concept has become increasingly accepted, particularly for the public sector in developing countries. Its appropriate application throughout the world remains a challenge for the future.

References

1. *IMS Marketletter,* 11 August 1986.

2. *World population prospects.* New York, UNDIESA, 1986 (Population Studies, No. 98).

3. *IMS Marketletter,* 9 June 1986.

4. UNITED NATIONS CONFERENCE ON TRADE AND DEVELOPMENT. *Handbook of international trade and development statistics, 1986. Supplement.* New York, UNCTAD, 1987.

5. MILLS, A. & WALKER, G.J.A. Drugs for the poor of the Third World: consumption and distribution. *Journal of tropical medicine and hygiene,* **86**: 139-145 (1983).

6. LASHMAN HALL, K. *Pharmaceuticals in the Third World: an overview.* Washington, DC, World Bank, 1986 (PHN Technical Note 86-31).

7. JANCLOES, M. ET AL. Financing urban primary health services. *Tropical doctor,* **15**: 98-104 (1985).

8. KASONGO PROJECT TEAM. Primary health care for less than a dollar a year. *World health forum,* **5**: 211-215 (1984).

9. UNITED NATIONS CENTRE ON TRANSNATIONAL CORPORATIONS. *Transnational corporations in the pharmaceutical industry of developing countries.* New York, UNCTC, 1983.

10. LAPORTE, J.R. ET AL. Drugs in the Spanish health system. *International journal of health services,* **14**: 635-648 (1984).

11. MEDAWAR, C. *Drugs and world health.* The Hague, International Organization of Consumers' Unions, 1984.

12. *The rational use of drugs. Report of the Conference of Experts, Nairobi, 25-29 November 1985.* Geneva, World Health Organization, 1987.

13. *SCRIP,* No. 1218, 1 August 1987.

14. REIS-ARNDT, E. A quarter of a century of pharmaceutical research. *Drugs made in Germany,* **30**: 105-112 (1987).

15. *Studies in drug utilization: methods and applications.* Copenhagen, WHO Regional Office for Europe, 1979 (European Series, No. 8).

16. STICKLER, G.B. Polypharmacy and poisons in pediatrics – the epidemic of overprescribing and ways to control it. *Advances in pediatrics,* **27**: 1-29 (1980).

17. BAKSAAS, I. Patterns in drug utilization. National and international aspects: antihypertensive drugs. *Acta medica scandinavica,* **683** (suppl.): 59-66 (1984).

18. O'BRIEN, B. *Patterns of European diagnosis and prescribing,* London, Office of Health Economics, 1984.

19. *The use of antibiotics worldwide. Report of Task Force 1.* Washington, DC, Fogarty International Center, National Institutes of Health, 1985.

20. AZARNOFF, D.L. Monitoring and control of physician prescribing are needed. In: Lasagna, L., ed., *Controversies in therapeutics.* Philadelphia, Saunders, 1980, pp. 534-541.

21. STEIN, C.M. ET AL. A survey of antibiotic use in Harare primary care clinic. *Journal of antimicrobial chemotherapy,* **14**: 149 (1984).

22. HOSSAIN, M.M. ET AL. Antibiotic use in a rural community in Bangladesh. *International journal of epidemiology,* **11**: 402-405 (1982).

23. CHONG, H.O.A. & LEE, D. Evaluación de terapía antimicrobiana en la sala de pediatría del hospital Manuel Amador Guerrero del systema integrado de salud de Colón. In: *The use of antibiotics worldwide, Report of Task Force 5.* Washington, DC, Fogarty International Center, National Institutes of Health, 1985.

24. PENG WEN WEI. Misuse of antibiotics, People's Republic of China. In: *The use of antibiotics worldwide, Report of Task Force 5*. Washington, DC, Fogarty International Center, National Institutes of Health, 1985.

25. KOPALA, L. The use of cimetidine in hospitalized patients. *Canadian family physician*, 30: 69-74 (1984).

26. *SCRIP*, No. 1189, 20 March 1987.

27. *SCRIP*, No. 1222, 15 July 1987.

28. HAYNES, R.B. ET AL. *Compliance in health care*. Baltimore, MD, Johns Hopkins University Press, 1979.

29. IGUN, U.A. Why we seek treatment here: retail pharmacy and clinical practice in Maiduguri, Nigeria. *Social science and medicine*, 24: 689-695 (1987).

30. *The growth of the pharmaceutical industry in developing countries: problems and prospects*. Vienna, United Nations Industrial Development Organization, 1978.

31. *A competitive assessment of the US pharmaceutical industry*. Washington, DC, United States Department of Commerce, 1986 (the figures are based on OECD data).

32. SCHAUMANN, L. ET AL. *A generics milestone*, Vol. I, Menlo Park, CA, SRI International, 1985.

33. JAMES, B.G. *The marketing of generic drugs*. London, Associated Business Press, 1982.

34. *SCRIP*, No. 1074, 5 February 1986.

35. SCHAUMANN, L. ET AL. *A generics milestone*, Vol. II, Menlo Park, CA, SRI International, 1985.

36. *SCRIP*, No. 914, 16 July 1984; No. 1198/9, 22-24 April 1987.

37. *SCRIP Yearbook*, Richmond, Surrey, SCRIP, 1987.

38. *IMS Marketletter*, 26 May 1986.

39. *Consumer reports*. Washington, DC, Federal Trade Commission, 1987.

40. *SCRIP*, No. 1039, 2 October 1985.

41. *SCRIP*, No. 1220, 8 July 1987.

42. *SCRIP*, No. 1166/7, 25 December 1986/1 January 1987.

43. *Changes and trends*. Richmond, Surrey, SCRIP, 1986.

44. CHEW, R. ET AL. *Pharmaceuticals in seven nations*. London, Office of Health Economics, 1985.

45. *SCRIP*, No. 1232, 17 August 1987.

46. *SCRIP*, No. 1032, 9 September 1985.

47. BARRAL, E. *Prospective et santé*, No. 36, Winter 1985/86, pp. 89-95.

48. *Pharmaceutical business opportunities with China: an analysis*. Richmond, Surrey, SCRIP, 1987.

49. *SCRIP*, No. 1171, 16 January 1987.

50. *SCRIP*, No. 1062, 23 December 1985.

51. *SCRIP*, No. 1205, 15 May 1987.

52. *Pharmaceuticals in developing countries*. London, Office of Health Economics, 1982.

53. FAUST, R.E. Envisioning the future of research and development. *Pharmaceutical executive*, September – October 1984.

54. *SCRIP*, No. 1081, 3 March 1986.

55. *SCRIP*, No. 1032, 9 September 1985.

56. *IMS Marketletter*, October 1984.

57. *SCRIP*, No. 1180, 18 February 1987.

58. Industria farmaceutica latinoamericana. *Alifar*, June 1986.

59. *IMS Marketletter*, 28 July 1986.

60. *SCRIP*, No. 1214, 17 June 1987.

61. *SCRIP*, No. 1224, 22 July 1987.

62. WHITE, E. Patents and the pharmaceutical industry – the other viewpoint. *SCRIP*, No. 1274, 15 January 1988.

63. *Policies for the production and marketing of essential drugs.* Washington, DC, Pan American Health Organization, 1984.

64. SILVERMAN, M. ET AL. Drug promotion: the Third World revisited. *International journal of health services*, 16: 659-667 (1986).

65. SZUBA, T.J. Drug promotion under the magnifying glass. *Journal of social and administrative pharmacy*, 4: 77-80 (1987).

66. *SCRIP*, No. 997, 8 May 1985.

67. *SCRIP*, No. 1231, 14 August 1987.

68. GOLDBERG, T. & DE VITO, C. A. The impact of state generic subtitution laws. In: Morgan, J.P. & Kagan, D.V., ed., *Society and medication: conflicting signals for prescribers and patients.* Lexington, MA, Lexington Books, 1983, pp. 99–110.

69. *SCRIP*, No. 1221, 10 July 1987.

70. *IMS Marketletter*, 5 May 1985.

Indicators used in Part II of this report

Policy

1 — There is no interest in a national pharmaceutical policy, or a national policy is under consideration.

2 — The national pharmaceutical policy is at an early stage.

3 — A national pharmaceutical policy exists.

Legislation

1 — A drug regulatory administration does not function and legislation is outdated.

2 — A drug regulatory administration is at an early stage (basic legislation and drug registration).

3 — A drug regulatory administration exists but is not fully functioning.

4 — There is an effective drug regulatory administration (evaluation of drugs, drug registration, quality control, inspection, product information).

Essential drugs list

1 — No essential drugs list exists or it is outdated.

2 — An essential drugs list exists by generic name for the public sector.

3 — An essential drugs list exists by generic name for the public sector and is used for drug management.

Procurement

1 — Procurement is direct or negotiated, prices are rather high.

2 — Procurement is by tender from multiple sources, takes quality and price into account, and medium prices are obtained.

3 — Procurement is by tender from multiple sources, takes quality and price into account, obtains good prices, and where financially and technically feasible, promotes local production.

Distribution

1 — The distribution system is deficient.

2 — A moderately good distribution system exists.

3 — A good distribution system exists.

Coverage

1 — Less than 30% of the population have regular access to essential drugs.

2 — 30–60% of the population have regular access to essential drugs.

3 — 60–90% of the population have regular access to essential drugs.

Quality assurance

1 — No quality assurance exists.

2 — Some quality assurance mechanisms exist, but there is no quality control laboratory.

3 — A quality assurance system, including a quality control laboratory, exists, but does not function adequately.

4 — A fully functioning quality assurance system, including a quality control laboratory, exists.

Information

1 — There is no organized provision of information to health workers and patients.

2 — The provision of information for health workers is semi-organized, and there is no systematic information for patients.

3 — A well-functioning system exists providing objective information on a regular basis to health workers about drug characteristics, safety, indications, contraindications, adverse reactions, dosage, costs, etc., with organized information for patients.

Manpower development

1 — Continuing education is not systematic.

2 — There is systematic continuing education for administrators, health care personnel, and quality control personnel.

Monitoring

1 — No monitoring mechanisms exist.

2 — Non-systematic monitoring mechanisms exist.

3 — Systematic mechanisms for drug monitoring exist, covering post-marketing surveillance and monitoring of adverse drug reactions.

Production

1 — No production takes place.

2 — Production of drugs from pharmaceutical chemicals takes place.

3 — Production of pharmaceutical chemicals takes place.

4 — There is research capability leading to discovery of new chemical entities.

Drug situation by country, 1986–87

	Coverage[a]	Policy	Legislation	Essential drugs list	Procure-ment	Distri-bution
Afghanistan	1	1	2	2	1	1
Algeria	3	3	3	3	3	3
Angola	1	2	1	3	2	1
Argentina	3	2	3	2	1	2
Bahamas	3	2	2	2	1	2
Bahrain	3	1	3	2	1	3
Bangladesh	1	3	3	2	2	1
Barbados	3	3	2	3	3	3
Benin	1	1	1	1	1	1
Bhutan	2	3	2	3	2	2
Bolivia	1	2	3	2	1	1
Botswana	3	2	1	3	2	3
Brazil	3	3	3	3	3	2
Burkina Faso	2	2	1	2	1	1
Burma	1	2	2	2	2	1
Burundi	2	2	2	2	2	2
Cameroon	1	1	1	1	1	1
Central African Republic	1	n.a.	n.a.	n.a.	n.a.	n.a.
Chad	1	n.a.	n.a.	n.a.	n.a.	n.a.
Chile	3	3	3	3	3	2
China	3	3	3	3	2	2
Colombia	2	2	3	2	1	1
Comoros	3	2	2	3	2	2
Costa Rica	3	3	4	3	2	2
Côte d'Ivoire	1	1	1	1	1	1
Cuba	3	3	4	3	3	3
Cyprus	3	2	4	3	3	3
Democratic Yemen	2	2	1	3	2	2
Djibouti	3	1	2	2	1	3
Dominica	2	1	1	2	2	2
Dominican Republic	2	2	3	2	2	1
Ecuador	2	2	3	2	2	1
Egypt	3	1	3	2	1	2
El Salvador	2	2	1	2	1	1
Equatorial Guinea	1	n.a.	n.a.	n.a.	n.a.	n.a.
Ethiopia	2	3	2	3	2	2
Fiji	3	n.a.	n.a.	2	1	2

n.a. = not available.
[a] 1 = group A; 2 = group B; 3 = group C.

Quality assurance	Information	Manpower development	Monitoring	Production	GDP per head (US$)	
3	1	1	1	2	164	Afghanistan
3	2	1	2	2	2 380	Algeria
1	1	1	1	2	341	Angola
3	2	1	2	4	2 230	Argentina
2	1	1	1	1	4 260	Bahamas
3	2	1	2	1	10 480	Bahrain
3	1	1	2	2	130	Bangladesh
3	2	1	2	1	4 340	Barbados
1	1	1	1	2	270	Benin
2	2	1	1	1	111	Bhutan
3	1	1	1	2	410	Bolivia
3	1	1	1	2	910	Botswana
4	2	1	2	3	1 710	Brazil
2	1	1	1	2	160	Burkina Faso
2	1	1	1	2	180	Burma
2	1	1	1	2	220	Burundi
1	1	1	1	2	810	Cameroon
n.a.	n.a.	n.a.	n.a.	n.a.	210	Central African Republic
n.a.	n.a.	n.a.	n.a.	2	150	Chad
4	2	1	2	2	1 710	Chile
3	2	1	1	4	224	China
3	2	1	2	2	1 370	Colombia
2	1	1	1	1	261	Comoros
3	2	2	3	2	1 210	Costa Rica
2	1	1	n.a.	2	610	Côte d'Ivoire
3	2	1	3	3	1 600	Cuba
4	2	2	3	2	3 590	Cyprus
1	2	2	1	2	510	Democratic Yemen
2	2	1	2	1	1 200	Djibouti
2	1	1	1	1	1 080	Dominica
3	1	1	1	2	960	Dominican Republic
3	1	1	1	2	1 220	Ecuador
3	2	1	2	3	720	Egypt
1	1	1	1	2	710	El Salvador
n.a.	n.a.	n.a.	n.a.	1	181	Equatorial Guinea
2	2	1	1	2	110	Ethiopia
2	1	1	1	1	1 840	Fiji

	Coverage[a]	Policy	Legislation	Essential drugs list	Procure- ment	Distri- bution
Gabon	3	n.a.	n.a.	2	1	2
Gambia	3	3	3	3	3	2
Ghana	2	2	2	2	2	2
Grenada	3	1	1	2	2	1
Guatemala	2	2	1	2	1	1
Guinea	1	2	1	2	1	1
Guinea-Bissau	2	2	1	3	2	2
Guyana	3	3	3	2	2	1
Haiti	2	1	1	2	1	1
Honduras	2	2	1	2	1	1
India	1	3	3	1	n.a.	2
Indonesia	2	3	3	3	3	2
Iran (Islamic Republic of)	3	3	4	3	3	3
Iraq	3	3	4	3	3	3
Jamaica	3	1	3	2	2	2
Jordan	3	1	3	2	3	2
Kenya	3	3	3	3	2	3
Kuwait	3	1	3	2	2	3
Lebanon	3	1	3	2	1	1
Lesotho	3	3	2	3	2	2
Liberia	1	1	1	2	1	1
Libyan Arab Jamahiriya	3	3	3	3	2	3
Madagascar	1	1	1	2	1	1
Malawi	2	2	1	3	3	2
Malaysia	3	2	3	3	2	2
Maldives	2	2	2	3	2	n.a.
Mali	1	2	2	2	1	1
Mauritania	1	1	2	1	1	1
Mauritius	3	2	3	3	3	3
Mexico	3	3	3	3	3	2
Morocco	2	1	3	2	2	2
Mozambique	2	3	3	3	3	1
Nepal	1	2	2	3	1	1
Nicaragua	3	3	3	3	3	1
Niger	2	1	1	1	1	2
Nigeria	1	2	3	2	1	1
Oman	3	1	3	1	2	2
Pakistan	2	1	3	2	2	2
Panama	3	2	3	3	2	2
Papua New Guinea	3	2	2	3	3	3
Peru	2	3	3	3	2	1
Philippines	1	2	2	2	1	1
Rwanda	1	1	1	2	1	1
Saint Lucia	3	2	1	3	2	2
Saudi Arabia	3	2	3	2	2	n.a.

n.a. = not available.

[a] 1 = group A; 2 = group B; 3 = group C.

Quality assurance	Information	Manpower development	Monitoring	Production	GDP per head (US$)	
n.a.	n.a.	n.a.	n.a.	1	3 480	Gabon
2	2	1	1	1	260	Gambia
3	1	1	1	2	350	Ghana
2	1	1	1	1	880	Grenada
3	1	1	1	2	1 120	Guatemala
1	1	1	1	2	300	Guinea
1	1	1	1	1	180	Guinea-Bissau
3	1	1	1	1	580	Guyana
1	1	1	1	2	320	Haiti
1	1	1	1	2	700	Honduras
3	1	1	2	4	260	India
4	2	1	3	3	540	Indonesia
3	2	1	3	3	2 500	Iran (Islamic Republic of)
4	2	1	3	3	2 218	Iraq
3	2	1	1	2	1 080	Jamaica
3	2	1	n.a.	2	1 710	Jordan
3	2	1	1	2	300	Kenya
4	n.a.	1	n.a.	2	15 410	Kuwait
3	2	1	1	2	970	Lebanon
3	2	1	1	1	530	Lesotho
1	1	1	1	2	470	Liberia
3	2	1	1	2	8 230	Libyan Arab Jamahiriya
1	1	1	1	2	270	Madagascar
2	1	1	1	2	210	Malawi
3	1	1	2	2	1 990	Malaysia
2	1	1	1	1	450	Maldives
1	1	1	1	2	210	Mali
1	1	1	1	1	450	Mauritania
2	2	1	1	2	1 100	Mauritius
4	2	1	2	3	2 060	Mexico
3	1	1	1	2	670	Morocco
3	2	1	1	2	200	Mozambique
2	1	1	1	2	160	Nepal
3	2	1	2	2	870	Nicaragua
3	1	1	1	2	190	Niger
3	1	1	1	2	770	Nigeria
3	1	1	1	1	6 230	Oman
3	1	1	1	3	380	Pakistan
3	2	1	2	2	2 100	Panama
2	1	1	1	1	760	Papua New Guinea
3	2	1	1	3	980	Peru
3	1	1	1	2	660	Philippines
2	1	1	1	2	270	Rwanda
2	2	1	1	1	1 130	Saint Lucia
3	2	1	2	2	10 740	Saudi Arabia

	Coverage[a]	Policy	Legislation	Essential drugs list	Procurement	Distribution
Senegal	1	1	1	1	1	1
Seychelles	3	3	2	3	2	2
Sierra Leone	2	2	1	2	1	1
Solomon Islands	3	n.a.	n.a.	2	1	2
Somalia	1	1	1	2	1	1
Sri Lanka	3	3	3	3	3	3
Sudan	1	2	2	3	2	1
Syrian Arab Republic	3	1	3	3	1	3
Thailand	2	3	3	3	3	3
Togo	2	1	1	2	2	2
Trinidad and Tobago	3	2	3	3	2	2
Tunisia	2	1	2	1	2	2
Uganda	2	2	2	3	2	1
United Republic of Tanzania	3	2	2	3	3	3
Uruguay	3	2	3	3	1	2
Vanuatu	3	n.a.	n.a.	2	1	n.a.
Venezuela	3	2	3	2	2	2
Viet Nam	2	2	1	3	2	2
Yemen	2	2	2	2	1	1
Zaire	2	1	2	2	1	2
Zambia	2	2	2	3	2	2
Zimbabwe	2	2	2	3	2	2

n.a. = not available.

[a] 1 = group A; 2 = group B; 3 = group C.

Quality assurance	Information	Manpower development	Monitoring	Production	GDP per head (US$)	
2	1	1	1	2	380	Senegal
2	2	1	2	1	2 430	Seychelles
1	1	1	1	2	300	Sierra Leone
2	1	1	1	1	680	Solomon Islands
1	1	1	1	2	260	Somalia
4	2	2	2	2	360	Sri Lanka
3	1	1	1	2	350	Sudan
4	2	1	2	2	1 870	Syrian Arab Republic
3	2	1	3	2	850	Thailand
2	1	1	1	2	292	Togo
3	2	1	1	1	7 140	Trinidad and Tobago
3	1	1	1	2	1 250	Tunisia
1	1	1	1	2	230	Uganda
2	2	1	1	2	280	United Republic of Tanzania
3	2	1	2	2	1 970	Uruguay
n.a.	1	1	1	1	389	Vanuatu
3	1	1	2	3	3 220	Venezuela
2	1	1	1	2	112	Viet Nam
2	1	1	1	2	510	Yemen
3	1	1	1	2	140	Zaire
2	2	1	1	2	470	Zambia
2	1	1	1	2	740	Zimbabwe

WHO publications may be obtained, direct or through booksellers, from:

ALGERIA: Entreprise nationale du Livre (ENAL), 3 bd Zirout Youcef, ALGIERS

ARGENTINA: Carlos Hirsch, SRL, Florida 165, Galerías Güemes, Escritorio 453/465, BUENOS AIRES

AUSTRALIA: Hunter Publications, 58A Gipps Street, COLLINGWOOD, VIC 3066.

AUSTRIA: Gerold & Co., Graben 31, 1011 VIENNA I

BAHRAIN: United Schools International, Arab Region Office, P.O. Box 726, BAHRAIN

BANGLADESH: The WHO Representative, G.P.O. Box 250, DHAKA 5

BELGIUM: *For books:* Office International de Librairie s.a., avenue Marnix 30, 1050 BRUSSELS. *For periodicals and subscriptions:* Office International des Périodiques, avenue Louise 485, 1050 BRUSSELS.

BHUTAN: *see* India, WHO Regional Office

BOTSWANA: Botsalo Books (Pty) Ltd., P.O. Box 1532, GABORONE

BRAZIL: Centro Latinoamericano de Informação em Ciencias de Saúde (BIREME), Organização Panamericana de Saúde, Sector de Publicações, C.P. 20381 - Rua Botucatu 862, 04023 SÃO PAULO, SP

BURMA: *see* India, WHO Regional Office

CAMEROON: Cameroon Book Centre, P.O. Box 123, South West Province, VICTORIA

CANADA: Canadian Public Health Association, 1335 Carling Avenue, Suite 210, OTTAWA, Ont. K1Z 8N8. (Tel: (613) 725–3769. Telex: 21–053–3841)

CHINA: China National Publications Import & Export Corporation, P.O. Box 88, BEIJING (PEKING)

DEMOCRATIC PEOPLE'S REPUBLIC OF KOREA: *see* India, WHO Regional Office

DENMARK: Munksgaard Export and Subscription Service, Nørre Søgade 35, 1370 COPENHAGEN K (Tel: + 45 1 12 85 70)

FIJI: The WHO Representative, P.O. Box 113, SUVA

FINLAND: Akateeminen Kirjakauppa, Keskuskatu 2, 00101 HELSINKI 10

FRANCE: Arnette, 2 rue Casimir-Delavigne, 75006 PARIS

GERMAN DEMOCRATIC REPUBLIC: Buchhaus Leipzig, Postfach 140, 701 LEIPZIG

GERMANY FEDERAL REPUBLIC OF: Govi-Verlag GmbH, Ginnheimerstrasse 20, Postfach 5360, 6236 ESCHBORN — Buchhandlung Alexander Horn, Kirchgasse 22, Postfach 3340, 6200 WIESBADEN

GREECE: G.C. Eleftheroudakis S.A., Librairie internationale, rue Nikis 4, 105-63 ATHENS

HONG KONG: Hong Kong Government Information Services, Publication (Sales) Office, Information Services Department, No. 1, Battery Path, Central, HONG KONG.

HUNGARY: Kultura, P.O.B. 149, BUDAPEST 62

ICELAND: Snaebjorn Jonsson & Co., Hafnarstraeti 9, P.O. Box 1131, IS-101 REYKJAVIK

INDIA: WHO Regional Office for South-East Asia, World Health House, Indraprastha Estate, Mahatma Gandhi Road, NEW DELHI 110002

IRAN (ISLAMIC REPUBLIC OF): Iran University Press, 85 Park Avenue, P.O. Box 54/551, TEHERAN

IRELAND: TDC Publishers, 12 North Frederick Street, DUBLIN 1 (Tel: 744835–749677)

ISRAEL: Heiliger & Co., 3 Nathan Strauss Street, JERUSALEM 94227

ITALY: Edizioni Minerva Medica, Corso Bramante 83–85, 10126 TURIN; Via Lamarmora 3, 20100 MILAN; Via Spallanzani 9, 00161 ROME

JAPAN: Maruzen Co. Ltd., P.O. Box 5050, TOKYO International, 100–31

JORDAN: Jordan Book Centre Co. Ltd., University Street, P.O. Box 301 (Al-Jubeiha), AMMAN

KENYA: Text Book Centre Ltd, P.O. Box 47540, NAIROBI

KUWAIT: The Kuwait Bookshops Co. Ltd., Thunayan Al-Ghanem Bldg, P.O. Box 2942, KUWAIT

LAO PEOPLE'S DEMOCRATIC REPUBLIC: The WHO Representative, P.O. Box 343, VIENTIANE

LUXEMBOURG: Librairie du Centre, 49 bd Royal, LUXEMBOURG

A/1/88